YOGA
THROUGH CHRIST
Via The Eight Limbs of Yoga

Sally Bassett, Ph.D.
Photographer Tricia Wright

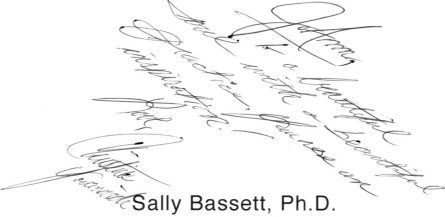

ISBN 978-1-63525-227-9 (Paperback)
ISBN 978-1-63525-228-6 (Digital)

Christian Faith Publishing, Inc.
296 Chestnut Street
Meadville, PA 16335
www.christianfaithpublishing.com

Printed in the United States of America

Dedication

To Olivia
Jesus loves you, this I know.

CONTENTS

INTRODUCTION

When I began practicing yoga on a regular basis in the early '90s, I questioned if this was a conflict with my Christian beliefs. Like most Westerners, I initially came to the mat because of the physical practice and all the benefits of calming the mind. The actual point of yoga, however, is to unite oneself with God. Yoga is not a religion, but a science or spiritual discipline that can provide helpful tools to strengthen one's own faith.

In time, I realized the yoga process, or the Eight Limbs of Yoga, provided a path to oneness with God. The first two limbs concentrate on external and internal values. Next come the postures to prepare the body physically to sit in prayer and meditation for long periods of time. Breath work is incorporated after the physical practice in order to calm the mind even further for meditation. It is then that the individual begins withdrawing from the senses, going inward to focus and pray, and eventually meditating and being with God.

In prayer, a person talks to God, and in meditation, one listens to God. Not to offend any Christian traditions, but I personally have found we do not "listen" enough. We go to church to praise God, but are we sincerely taking the time to feel His presence and listen?

It is with great respect and faith that I have prayed to God on the banks of the Ganga River in India with hundreds of spiritual individuals, listened to the beliefs from our own Native American Indians in South Dakota, and visited cathedrals across the globe and lit candles too numerous to count. As a Christian, I have meditated in Muslim prayer rooms in airports throughout the world, sung gospel songs around campfires with rural women in Uganda, sat with monks in silence across Asia, and learned about religions wherever I have traveled.

When I step on the yoga mat, I experience a deep sense of peace and a closer spiritual connection to myself and to God. When I follow the Eight Limbs of Yoga, it takes me to a deeper level. One of my favorite quotes by Rumi resonates with me even more, "Seek the path that demands your whole being." This path has brought me closer to God than I could ever imagine.

The goal of yoga is to experience the spiritual presence of God. In *Prayer of Heart and Body* by Thomas Ryan, he explained, "When the science of yoga was brought to the West, a discernment was obviously made that the potential market would be greater if the physical health benefits were stressed, and the religious and spiritual ends of the practice were allowed to fade in the background." Ryan began meditating because he wanted a relationship of intimacy with God. He found it there, and so can you.

In his book, *The Wisdoms of Jesus and the Yoga Siddhas*, Marshall Govindan revealed "that recent research by independent scholars has uncovered many details about what Jesus taught, which when compared to the teachings of classical yoga, indicates close similarities both in what he practiced, and what he realized."

Paramahansa Yogananda, author of *The Autobiography of a Yogi*, is renowned as "the Father of Yoga in the West" and one of the key spiritual figures of our time. He believed that every seeker could know God not through mere belief but by direct experience via yoga meditation. God can be known, not as a theological concept but as an actual personal experience. The goal of this book is to show individuals exactly how they can have a closer relationship with God… one step at a time.

I pray with time that many people can become even stronger in their faith with Christ through the Eight Limbs of Yoga.

The Four Main Paths of Yoga

Yoga through Christ embraces the full range of spiritual paths to one's union with God. As the practioner becomes adept in the four pathways, they will begin to flow together. Mahatma Gandhi believed, "Truth is One, Paths are Many."

Raja Yoga is the most structured or royal path and includes the eight limbed progression. This was codified by Patanjali about 1500–2000 years ago in the famous ancient yoga text entitled the *Yoga Sutras*. This is considered the original textbook of classical yoga, and though it is thousands of years old, it is still relevant today. Raja yoga is the path that leads to union with God through the mental mastery of the mind, body, and breath. It calls upon the physical and mental discipline of the poses of Hatha Yoga.

Bhakti Yoga is the path of devotion and intense love for God. Patanjali was a *bhakti*—a lover of God. It is practiced by most major religions through worship, prayer, singing, and rituals. It seeks salvation through love and prayer.

Jnana Yoga is the path of wisdom through the study of ancient texts, including self-study. This path is an on on-going, never-ending search for deeper understanding through the acquisition of knowledge.

Karma Yoga is the path of selfless service to others. It takes yoga off the mat and into the world. Because those acts are done without attachment to the results, it gives all credit to God as the Doer. The thought behind it is, "Just be good and do good." It is a simple path when there is love.

In another ancient yoga text, the Bhagavad-Gita states, "Work alone is your privilege, never the fruits thereof. Never let the fruits of action be your motive, and never cease to work. Work in the name of the Lord, abandoning selfish desires. Be not affected by success or failure. This equipoise is called yoga."

Mother Teresa's life demonstrated a great example of karma yoga. She once said to find peace, we just need to take a simple path. Below is her own prayer that she followed:

The fruit of silence is Prayer.
The fruit of prayer is Faith.
The fruit of faith is Love.
The fruit of love is Service.
The fruit of service is Peace.

The purpose of these four main types of yoga is to bring the individual closer to God through meditation, religious devotions, study, and selfless service to others.

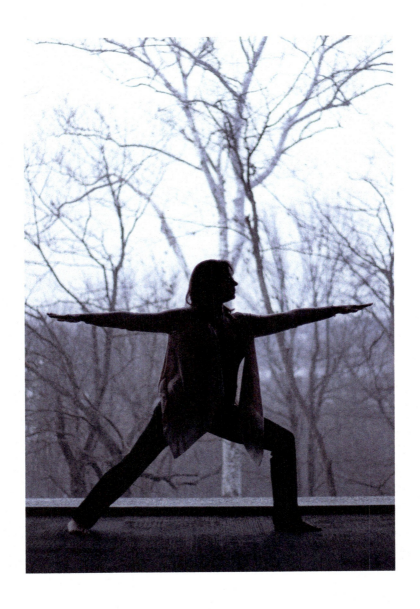

CHAPTER 1

The Eight Limbs of Yoga

Our success-oriented society continues to search for ways to achieve total well-being even in the midst of a stressful and fast-paced lifestyle. The practice of yoga offers a limitless wellspring of healing and vitality for people of all backgrounds, age groups, religions, and physiques. Yoga reunites our outer worldly existence with that deeper inner experience of who we really are. It brings all parts of our being into harmony—the mental, emotional, physical, and spiritual sides.

The real purpose of yoga is for an individual to connect to a higher power through mind, body, and spirit. A pioneer for Christian yoga, Susan Bordenkircher, wrote, "Yoga is a universal practice thousands of years old, predating Hinduism, and was not designed specific to any religion. It is considered a framework or guideline to direct people toward greater spiritual growth and physical health."

In 2004, *The Los Angeles Times* published an article about Yogananda and verified, "Yoga is one of the world's oldest and most systematic religious paths to achieving oneness with God."

Well-known and beloved yogi, BKS Iyengar, explained, "Nowhere in the ancient texts is it said that yoga is only to be practiced by the Hindus. Yoga is a universal culture." Yoga is meant for all humanity. A yogi's actions are performed with purity and divinity. Yoga instills in the person to be Christ-like. Yoga starts with a code of conduct, in which each individual is challenged to develop. The essence of a true religion is the same as yoga, which is the linking back, specifically, linking the soul of its follower back to its original source: God.

Most people think yoga is only a physical practice. In fact, within the Eight Limbs of Yoga, only one limb is about the postures (exercise poses). No one element of these eight limbs takes precedence over the other because all contribute to the structural foundation of yoga.

It has been documented, even though somewhat controversial, that during the unaccounted years of Jesus's life from approximately age fourteen to twenty-eight, he might have traveled to India and Tibet for meditation. These ancient records were supposedly discovered and copied in the Himis Monastery in Tibet by a Russian traveler, Nicholas Notovitch, who published his notes in 1984 under the title, *The Unknown Life of Jesus Christ*.

The following illustration of the Eight Limbed Path of Yoga briefly explains how yoga provides guidelines for individuals to become better human beings by connecting to God.

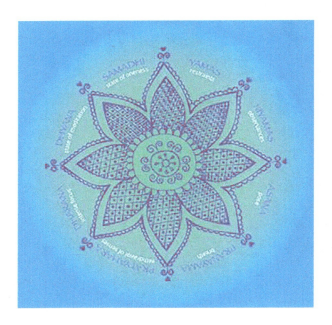

Yoga: The Eight Limbed Path

1. Yamas - Social Observances/Restraints
   * Nonviolence
   * Truthfulness
   * Non-stealing
   * Moderation
   * Non-attachment

2. Ni-Yamas - Internal Observances
   * Cleanliness or purity
   * Contentment
   * Burning desire
   * Self-study
   * Surrender to God

3. Asana - Poses
4. Pranayama - Breath Control
5. Pratyahara - Withdrawal of the Senses
6. Dharana – Concentration and Prayer
7. Dhyana – Meditation and Being with God
8. Samadhi - Oneness with God

Understanding the Eight Limbs of Yoga is vital to the practice and study of yoga. Imagine the eight limbs as the arms and legs of a body. Each limb is connected to one another through the central body of yoga, and whatever limb of practice we focus upon inevitably causes the other limbs to grow stronger as well.

Yoga is called a "practice" because it is a lifelong journey. Everyone who approaches the practice of yoga with an open heart, learns from this ancient five-thousand-plus-year-old practice. In time, with practice and faith, the progression of the eight limbs of yoga will bring oneness with God.

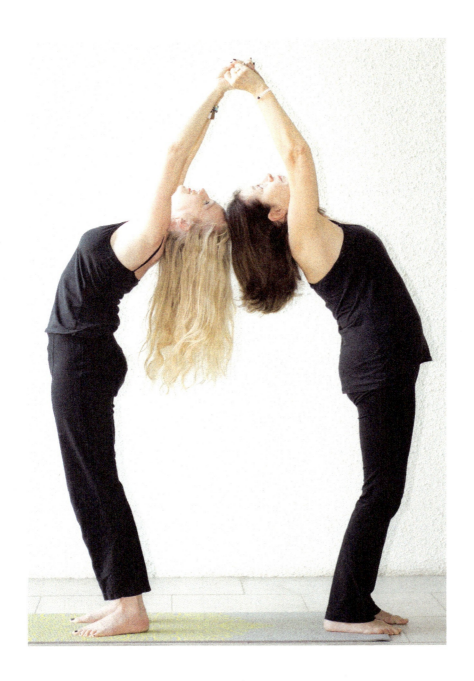

CHAPTER 2

The First Limb of Yoga: Social Observances (Yamas)

Before someone ever gets on a mat, a yogi should understand that yoga is not just a physical practice. It is a life practice. It begins with five social observances. These five values focus on moral, ethical, and spiritual principles. These restraints are nonviolence, truth, non-stealing, moderation, and non-attachment.

As an instructor of yoga teacher trainings, at the beginning of our first class, I often ask new students to sit to the right of their mat and to commit to these five principles for living harmoniously in the world.

The five external disciplines restraints are as follows:

- ***Nonviolence (Ahimsa)***

The practice of nonviolence (ahimsa) includes physical, mental, and emotional kindness towards others, as well as, one's self. It is nonviolence in thought, word, and deed. In theory, by practicing this discipline, a person should eventually be able to replace hatred with love. To accomplish this goal requires a lot of work and self-discipline. Eliminating any physically abuse, of course, is the first step to do. After that, controlling one's self to avoid hurting others with words. Next, an individual would need to recognize subtle actions that hurt others, such as gossiping, lying, cussing, and rudeness. Those who practice ahimsa learn to control their negative thoughts and attitudes about others and themselves. Learn to **THINK**; in other words, asking if an action is True, Helpful, Improves, Necessary, and Kind?

It can be easy to become addicted to anger, gossip, and criticism. When you become aware of it, let it go. This awareness and gentleness in thought, action, and speech should include all beings, including yourself (and even bugs). Any violence falls away in the presence of such unconditional love generated through the practice of nonviolence. Mother Teresa once eloquently stated, "If you judge people, you have no time to love them."

To begin practicing ahimsa, a good recommendation is to follow international yoga teacher Seane Corn's, advice: *"Ignore the story, see the soul."* Recognize there is a value and purpose for every person in life—and maybe especially in your life. I try to remind my yoga students of this prior to the holidays. Each of us has an "Aunt Bea" or a certain peer from work that you need to say to yourself, "Ignore the story and see the soul."

In his book, *The Heart and Science of Yoga*, Leonard Perlmutter wrote, "True heart-centered yoga means swimming against the tide of our culture and the habits of a lifetime to rely on the power of love and eternal wisdom that already reside within you."

There is no way to find stillness of the mind if harboring anger, resentment, or aversion. A person cannot love God and dislike anyone.

Jesus encourages his followers to love their enemies. The God of peace became human and walked the earth making peace, speaking for peace, and acting for peace so that all humanity might live in peace with each other and with God. Jesus embodies nonviolence. When in doubt, ask yourself the question "What Would Jesus Do?" WWJD is a great acronym to remember in tough situations.

+ **Scripture References for Nonviolence (Ahimsa)**

"But I say to you, love your enemies and pray for those who harass you so that you will be acting as children of your Father who is in heaven. He makes the sun rise on both the evil and the good and sends rain on both the righteous and the unrighteous" (Matthew 5:44–45)

"Happy are people who make peace, because they will be called God's children" (Matthew 5:9).

"Whatever you do, whether in speech or action, do it all in the name of the Lord Jesus and give thanks to God the Father through Him" (Colossians 3:17)

"Act wisely toward outsiders, making the most of the opportunity. Your speech should always be gracious and sprinkled with insight so that you may know how to respond to every person" (Colossians 4:5–6).

"Don't judge, so that you won't be judged. You'll receive the same judgment you give. Whatever you deal out will be dealt out to you" (Matthew 7:1–2).

"Let go of anger and leave rage behind! Don't get upset—it will only lead to evil. Because evildoers will be eliminated, but those who hope in the Lord—they will possess the land" (Psalm 37:8–9).

"Do you love life; do you relish the chance to enjoy good things? Then you must keep your tongue from evil and keep your lips from speaking lies! Turn away from evil! Do good! Seek peace and go after it!" (Psalm 34:12–14)

Letters from Prison (Ahimsa)

Correspondence between John, an inmate in a northern Indiana prison, and I began in the winter of 2012. After two incredible weeks in India, I was on my thirty-hour journey back to the States. While I was there, one of our yoga teachers handed me a letter that had been mailed to our yoga center in Indianapolis and had been meaning to give it to me.

It was from a man incarcerated in prison and was seeking some answers regarding the deeper side of yoga. Below is his letter and my response.

January 2012

To whom it may concern,

I am writing to you in regards to literature relating to the spiritual side of yoga. I have been practicing yoga for about ten months now and find a release from my present situation which nothing else can bring. I have a subscription to "Yoga Journal" which gives me some intellectual understanding but I need more. My first book on yoga was "Light on Yoga." It mentioned the BagavaGita and its poetic style of writing. My aunt is the one responsible for sending me such great material, but she is limited. Wanting to understand yoga in a deeper sense, I asked for more books. She then sent me "How Yoga Works" and the "Yoga Journal" subscription.

As you can see, I'm presently incarcerated and fortunately have plenty of time to read. LOL. I don't plan on being incarcerated forever, but while I'm here I would like to devote my time to understanding this wonderful thing called Yoga. I'm twenty-six years old with a background in martial arts, so flexibility (asanas) has come to me with ease. Unfortunately, Christianity is hindering me from opening my mind to the spiritual side of yoga, and I find the articles in Yoga Journal to be a little mushy for me—a "convict." LOL. Is there someone to correspond with me and help me answer questions I might come across in the future?

In closing and, in short, I guess I'm asking for some assistance or guidance. If you or this yoga center is able to help me on my way then I would be forever indebted to you. Thank you very much for your time or consideration on this matter.

Sincerely,
John

Saturday, March 10, 2012... I replied,

Dear John,

Thank you for your letter to Peace through Yoga (PTY) inquiring about the spiritual side of yoga. First, let me apologize for not writing sooner. I am currently 39,000 feet high in an aircraft returning from India. Your letter was given to me while I was in India by one of our yoga teachers at PTY. She had been carrying it around for quite a while meaning to give to me. Maybe it was not meant for me to reply to you until after this two-week journey to Rishikesh, the yoga capital of the world.

Second, it is awesome that you have discovered yoga and are reading "Yoga Journal," Iyengar's "Light on Yoga," and anything else you can find. Your current circumstances just might give you the opportunity to truly explore yoga and meditation in a way that many people cannot—or say they can't find the time. Take advantage of it! After two weeks on the Ganges River, there is nothing like being able to practice yoga fully—mind, body, and spirit, many hours a day.

Most Westerners come to yoga for the physical exercise. That's okay—it gets you into your body as well as mentally become focused. It sounds like you have the flexibility, strength, and endurance that most people seek during their physical practice of yoga. Your questions at this stage, wondering about the spiritual side of yoga, are natural.

I, too, am a strong Christian and had these same questions when I started practicing on a regular basis twelve to thirteen years ago. I soon signed up for Yoga Teacher Training. During that year, each student was required to do individual research on a subject or area of their choice. My research was entitled "Yoga through Christ."

Yoga is definitely not a religion. It is a science that can actually bring you to a deeper religious practice regardless what you believe. Don't let that scare you. Yoga was developed over 5000 years ago with the physical postures (asanas, as you know) being such a very small part of it. It was practiced to still the mind.

There couldn't be a better time for yoga to be growing in the United States with all the multi-tasking we do and the "monkey-mind" never ceasing. Through concentration and meditation, you can also have a closer relationship with God than ever before.

I like simple so let me end by sharing the Eight Limbs of Yoga. Try to learn and truly understand each Limb. If you aren't doing pranayama as part of your practice (breath work), it will be a great place to start.

- *Yamas – the five ethical principles you observe before ever getting on the mat: nonviolence (ahimsa), non-stealing (asteya), non-attachment or non-greediness (aparigraha), moderation (brahmacharya), and truthfulness (satya)*
- *Ni-Yamas—the five observances: cleanliness, contentment, burning desire to achieve goals, self-study, and surrendering to God*
- *Asanas—yogic poses: the hundreds of physical postures that get your mind and body ready for meditation*
- *Pranayama—breath control for cleansing, balancing, and calming. Just focusing on your breath is meditation*
- *Pratyahara—withdrawal of the senses*

- *Dharana—concentration*
- *Dhyana—meditation*
- *Samadhi—connection to a higher source*

Once again, just take a little bit at a time. It is called a "yoga practice" because it is a lifelong journey of learning.

Enclosed is a great international magazine that has an article on the Eight Limbs as well as the Chakras. If you are not familiar with the seven Chakras, I think you will enjoy learning about these energy sources in your body that can be blocked. I personally love bringing the Chakras into my teaching.

This past week I read an incredible book, "The Journey Home—Autobiography of an American Swami." I will try to track down a copy for you. In the meantime, take care of yourself and enjoy discovering yoga. There is nothing like it.

Namaste—which means the light in me recognizes and respects the light within you.

Sally from Peace through Yoga

The correspondence continued and was an extraordinary exchange of yoga philosophy and applying that to everyday life. John eventually began taking yoga teacher training by mail with me for over a year. During his training, John offered yoga and meditation classes to fellow prisoners. Below are segments of letters from John on nonviolence.

August 2:

Every time I teach yoga now in prison I hand out the five blue strips you gave me at the beginning of every class and have them read aloud. For instance: AHIMSA—an excellent form of nonviolence is selfless love and the most extreme form of violence is hatred. This day I will keep my actions focused on a loving awareness. I will hold an attitude of loving kindness to myself and to others. I will be aware of the fear, anger, selfishness, or other uncomfortable mental states without being carried away into an aggressive expression of the energy.

August 16:

You spoke about how it boggles your mind when I speak of the prison gang and violence. Well, let me tell you about a recent occurrence with my pride. Recently I was offended by the way this black dude spoke to me, and I reacted without being present. Sally, I violated nonviolence! Yet there was something holding me back because I hesitated. This hesitation resulted in him getting the upper hand. I didn't get hurt at all, but my pride was crushed and every time I look at him I regret the hesitation. I battle with the fact that I know beyond a reasonable doubt that I can beat him up. On top of that I have everyone who has seen me fight tell me things like, "I know you spared him." I never threw one punch or kick and now this dude thinks he beat me up. I breathe in the pride of his and mine and devour it in my furnace (tapas). Can't remember the name of this pranayama off the top of my head. Pretty sure you have mentioned it. So in reality I still have a temper with an ability to express it, which is something I work on daily. My mantra is "peace" (inhale) and "love" (exhale).

• *Truth (Satya)*

This discipline is about truthfulness in speech, actions, and thoughts. It is the avoidance of all lies, exaggeration and pretense. Satya is the practice of being honest in one's life. First and foremost, it must be in harmony with nonviolence. Those who emote honesty use positive wording to avoid hurting others while still being sincere and straightforward. Honesty is difficult to put into practice because sometimes the truth can hurt, yet, being honest and considerate of others feelings is still important to establish positive relationships. It is about living in harmony with integrity.

Since yoga is centered on creating a unity between mind, body, and spirit, it is important to ask yourself, "Am I practicing yoga from my real and honest self, or from an ego-centered place?"

One of the more famous verses about truth in the Bible is when Jesus declared, "*I am the way, the truth, and the life.*" (John 14:6). Jesus is truth, and Jesus is also the Word (John 1:1, 14). Knowing what the Bible says about truth and not hiding God's word in our heart helps us to know when we are listening to the Voice of Truth. Remember, it is more powerful to live truth than to preach it.

+ **Scripture Reference on Truth (Satya)**

"Little children, let's not love with words or speech but with action and truth. This is how we will know that we belong to the truth and reassure our hearts in God's presence" (1 John 3:18–19).

"Jesus said to the Jews who believed in him, 'You are truly my disciples if you remain faithful to my teaching. Then you will know the truth, and the truth will set you free" (John 8:31–32).

"God's goal is for us to become mature adults—to be fully grown, measured by the standard of the fullness of Christ. As a result, we aren't supposed to be infants any longer who can be tossed and blown around by every wind that comes from teaching with deceitful scheming and the tricks people play to deliberately mislead others. Instead, by speaking the truth with love, let's grow in every way into Christ" (Ephesians 4:13–15).

"Jesus answered, 'I am the way, the truth, and the life." (John 14:6).

"The Lord detests false lips, but he favors those who do what is true" (Proverbs 12:22).

"However, when the Spirit of Truth comes, he will guide you in all truth. He won't speak on his own, but will say whatever he hears and will proclaim to you what is to come" (John 16:13).

"Therefore, after you have gotten rid of lying, *each of you must tell the truth to your neighbor* because we are parts of each other in the same body" (Ephesians 4:25).

- ### *Non-stealing (Asteya)*

Non-stealing asks that we take only what is offered and use only what we need. This can be practiced in the realms of material resources, intellectual material, and respect for others' time and energy. This concept can be applied to many different aspects of life as well. One example is eating. It means to eat what we need versus eating what we want, which in turn, actually contributes to our own health.

Non-stealing is also about honoring boundaries, not coveting or being jealous. It is the freedom from craving or desiring what others have, giving credit where it is due, and not taking even ideas or attention from another.

Stealing is often due to a lack of faith in ourselves that we cannot create what we actually need. There is an insecurity, often even a worry that we do not have as much as others. As a result, we sometimes tend to become greedy and keep things for ourselves rather than share and give back to others.

Yoga teaches the practioner that once they surrender their desires for something, a true wealth will come on its own in many different ways. We give purely because of our gratitude for having received. Nothing truly belongs to us in the first place.

+ Scripture Reference for Non-Stealing (Asteya)

"Thieves should no longer steal. Instead, they should go to work, using their hands to do good so that they will have something to share with whoever is in need" (Ephesians 4:28).

"Do not steal" and "Do not covet" (Exodus 20:15 and 17a).

"Don't trust in violence; don't set false hopes in robbery. When wealth bears fruit, don't set your heart on it" (Psalm 62:10).

"So pay everyone what you owe them. Pay the taxes you owe, pay the duties you are charged, give respect to those you should respect, and honor those you should honor" (Romans 13:7).

"Give to Caesar what belongs to Caesar and to God what belongs to God" (Matthew 22:21).

"If you have persuaded yourself that you are: a guide for the blind; a light to those who are in darkness; an educator of infants (since you have the full content of knowledge and truth in the Law); then why don't you who are teaching others teach yourself? If you preach, 'No stealing,' do you steal?" (Romans 2:19–21).

"This is love: that we live according to his commands. This is the command that you heard from the beginning: live in love" (2 John 1:6).

• *Moderation (Brahmacharya)*

Moderation (also referred to as sexual purity) means self-restraint in order to use that energy toward other spiritual and devotional practices. The word translates to "walk with God." By following this principle, one can gain a greater sense of happiness and moral strength. Yoga is also about maintaining a balance. This means people should practice moderation in all of their activities—watching TV, shopping, surfing the internet, drinking caffeine, eating chocolate... (The last one is the hardest for me). When people work to satisfy their senses, they have less time and energy to direct toward meditation. Moderation is a commitment to using energy wisely—neither suppressing nor overindulging.

You do not have to be detached from society to achieve this spiritual oneness with God. Jesus himself was celibate and practiced poverty, meditation, and nonviolence. But he also served people daily, communicated with the masses, and drank wine moderately.

+ **Scripture References for Moderation (Brahmacharya)**

"Therefore, if you were raised with Christ, look for the things that are above where Christ is sitting at God's right side. Think about the things above and not things on earth" (Colossians 3:1–2).

"So be careful to live your life wisely, not foolishly. Take advantage of every opportunity because these are evil times. Because of this, don't be ignorant, but understand the Lord's will. Don't get drunk on wine, which produces depravity. Instead, be filled with the Spirit in the following ways: speak to each other with psalms, hymns, and spiritual songs; sing and make music to the Lord in your hearts; always give thanks to God the Father for everything in the name of our Lord Jesus Christ" (Ephesians 5:15–20).

"The grace of God has appeared, bringing salvation to all people. It educates us so that we can live sensible, ethical, and godly lives right now by rejecting ungodly lives and the desires of this world" (Titus 2:11–12).

"Avoid sexual immorality! Every sin that a person can do is committed outside the body, except those engaging in sexual immorality commit sin against their own bodies. Or don't you know that your body is a temple of the Holy Spirit who is in you? Don't you know that you have the Holy Spirit from God, and you don't belong to yourselves?" (I Corinthians 6:18–19).

"You were called to freedom, brothers and sisters; only don't let this freedom be an opportunity to indulge your selfish impulses, but serve each other through love. All the Law has been fulfilled in a single statement: *Love your neighbor as yourself*" (Galatians 5:13–14).

"Everyone who competes practices self-discipline in everything. The runners do this to get a crown of leaves that shrivel up and die, but we do it to receive a crown that never dies" (I Corinthians 9:25).

"Eating too much honey isn't good, nor is it appropriate to seek honor. A person without self-control is like a breached city, one with no walls" (Proverbs 25:27–28).

- ### *Non-attachment (Aparigraha)*

The final principle of the first limb of yoga (social restraints) is non-attachment or non-greediness. This particular principle emphasizes being truly happy with what we have. It is not about searching for that happiness through possessions or another individual. Practicing non-attachment will eventually lead to having no expectations in life that could hinder contentment and happiness with life and ourselves.

Non-attachment should not be misunderstood as indifference. The secret is that any desire without any personal or selfish motive will never bind us. Selfless desire has absolutely no expectations, so it knows no disappointment no matter what the results. By renouncing worldly things, we possess the most important sacred property: peace.

For example, hoarding could be considered a violation of this practice. When people hoard, they are keeping things for themselves that they really do not need instead of giving to charity, sharing with others, or eliminating waste.

Non-attachment teaches us to simplify and let go, even of our concepts and the need to "have things our way." If someone really wants to be greedy, may they be greedy in serving others.

Sogyal Rinpoche, author of *The Tibetan Book of Living and Dying*, once explained, "Freedom does not come from acquisition. It comes from letting go." Buddha considered attachment to be a root cause of suffering. The Bible further clarifies, "You are my Lord. Apart from you I have nothing good" (Psalms 16:2).

Sometimes we have certain habits or things that we think we cannot give up, but with reflection, we can see how they are binding us. Below are two ways to explore non-attachment:

- *Get rid of clothes that have not been worn in two years.* The rule of thumb used to be a year, but let's go with two years. Simply identify what is truly being used and eliminate what isn't. It will make life easier knowing what is in the closet is being used and will enable making the most of what is owned.

- *Reduce the amount of knickknacks and clutter.* Somewhere along the line of economic growth people started buying items just to put on shelves for decoration. These "things" may have lots of memories or be just fillers picked up at a flea market. It can be hard parting with "things," but try this simple suggestion. Get a bag, walk around the house, and look at each item. If it is something that hasn't been looked at for years and it is gathering dust, ask, "Is it time to part ways?" So, put it in the bag and continue exploring the other rooms. Once the bag is filled, take it to Goodwill or the Salvation Army. (I always have a sack in the pantry for clothes and knickknacks ready to be donated.)

May these two simple suggestions teach us to really examine our lifestyles and see what needs to stay and what needs to be on the way out.

+ Scripture References for Non-Attachment (Aparigraha)

"Stop collecting treasures for your own benefit on earth, where moth and rust eat them and where thieves break in and steal them. Instead, collect treasures for yourselves in heaven, where moth and rust don't eat them and where thieves don't break in and steal them. Where your treasure is, there your heart will be also" (Matthew 6: 19–21).

"I say to the Lord, 'You are my Lord. Apart from you, I have nothing good" (Psalm 16:2).

"Don't be afraid, little flock, because your Father delights in giving you the kingdom. Sell your possessions and give to those in need. Make for yourselves wallets that don't wear out—a treasure in heaven that never runs out. No thief comes near there, and no moth destroys. Where your treasure is, there your heart will be too" (Luke 12:32–34).

"Actually, godliness is a great source of profit when it is combined with being happy with what you already have. We didn't bring anything into the world and so we can't take anything out of it" (I Timothy 6:6–7).

"Peace I leave with you. My peace I give you. I give to you not as the world gives. Don't be troubled or afraid" (John 14:27).

"The actions that are produced by selfish motives are obvious, since they include sexual immorality, moral corruption, doing whatever feels good, idolatry, drug use and casting spells, hate, fighting, obsession, losing your temper, competitive opposition, conflict, selfishness, group rivalry, jealousy, drunkenness, partying, and other things like that. I warn you as I have already warned you, that those who do these kinds of things won't inherit God's kingdom. But the fruit of the Spirit is love, joy, peace, patience, kindness, goodness, faithfulness, gentleness, and self-control. There is no law against these things" (Galatians 5: 19–23).

"Whoever keeps these commands and teaches people to keep them will be called great in the kingdom of heaven" (Matthew 5:19b).

Practicing the five social observances is a difficult and challenging task, but when people truly make the effort, it can help them live happier, healthier, and holier lives.

****

Exercises:

1. Write what each of the five social observances/restraints mean to you.
2. Choose one that you are committed to for self-improvement as a yogi.
3. How do you practice and not practice nonviolence?

4. Think of a time when you exaggerated the truth and if it was needed?
5. What is the hardest thing about "non-attachment" for you?
6. Write about three people who have been major influences in your life and why?
7. Write a letter to someone you want to forgive or be forgiven.
8. Pick one negative aspect in your life that causes a block to joy and peace, such as anger, jealousy, impatience, etc. Develop a written plan to eradicate it from your life.
9. Add three new scripture verses for each social observance.

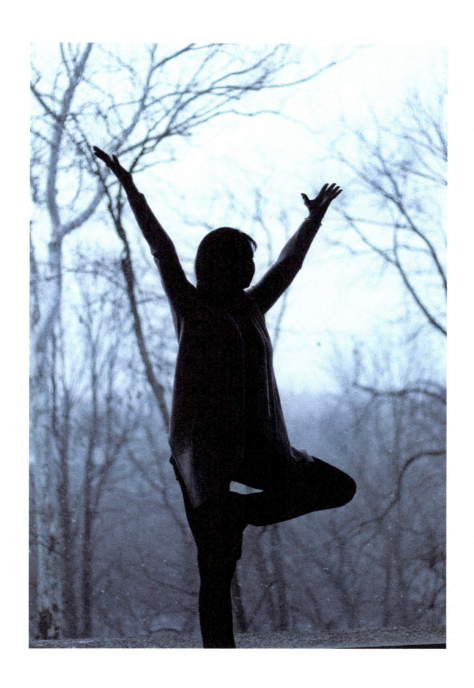

CHAPTER 3

The Second Limb of Yoga – Individual Observances (Ni-Yamas)

As previously stated, the Eight Limbs of Yoga act as guidelines on how to live a meaningful and purposeful life. Ni-yamas, or individual practices, is the second limb and consists of five principles: cleanliness, contentment, burning desire, self-study, and surrender to God. This is the inner work that teaches us to cultivate a closer relationship with God.

- *Cleanliness (Saucha)*

Cleanliness and purity, or Saucha, involves maintaining cleanliness in body, mind, and environment so that we can experience a higher quality of life. When we eat healthy foods, such as the recommended amounts of vegetables, fruits, proteins, carbohydrates, and dairy, the body starts to function more smoothly. When we read books that elevate our consciousness; when we see movies that inspire us; when we associate with kind people, we are feeding our mind and souls in a way that nourishes our own peacefulness. When we create a home environment that is cozy but simple, we are not constantly distracted by the things that surround us.

Saucha enables us to pursue and keep good healthy habits physically, emotionally, mentally, and environmentally.

+ Scripture Reference for Cleanliness (Saucha)

"Happy are people who have pure hearts, because they will see God" (Matthew 5:8).

"Create a clean heart for me, God; put a new, faithful spirit deep inside me!" (Psalm 51:10).

"My dear friends, since we have these promises, let's cleanse ourselves from anything that contaminates our body or spirit so that we make our holiness complete in the fear of God" (2 Corinthians 7:1).

"He saved us because of his mercy, not because of righteous things we had done. He did it through the washing of new birth and the renewing by the Holy Spirit, which God poured out upon us generously through Jesus Christ our Savior" (Titus 3:5–6).

"Wash! Be clean! Remove your ugly deeds from my sight. Put an end to such evil" (Isaiah 1:16).

"If we claim, e don't have any sin,' we deceive ourselves and the truth is not in us. But if we confess our sins, he is faithful and just to forgive us our sins and cleanse us from everything we've done wrong" (I John 1:8–9).

"I will sprinkle clean water on you, and you will be cleansed of all your pollution. I will cleanse you of all your idols. I will give you a new heart and put a new spirit in you. I will remove your stony heart from your body and replace it with a living one" (Ezekiel 36:25–26).

• *Contentment (Santosha)*

Contentment, or Santosha, is the ability to feel satisfied within the present moment. It is a sign that we are at peace with whatever stage of growth we are in and with the circumstances we find ourselves. It is also a choice. We can remain calm and open with success or failure or get depressed when things don't go the way we would like.

Yoga philosophy helps us to have no illusions about true happiness. It can be ours, but on the condition that we work to purify our minds as well as our bodies. To be truly happy, every individual must have a stable point which can hold them in place permanently. For most, this is their faith. Even in the bad times, they know God is there, holding them in safe harbor.

Happiness is not found in things. No person on earth can control life. It is too unpredictable. One day a person can be wealthy, the next day the economy could fall and take away everything.

True happiness and peace comes from faith in God. This can be experienced through a successful practice of yoga, for true happiness can only come from following the spiritual path.

+ Scripture References on Contentment (Santosha)

"Therefore, I say to you, don't worry about your life, what you'll eat or what you'll drink, or about your body, what you'll wear. Isn't life more than food and the body more than clothes? Look at the birds in the sky. They don't sow seed or harvest grain, or gather crops into barns. Yet your heavenly Father feeds them. Aren't you worth much more than they are? Who among you by worrying can add a single moment to your life?" (Matthew 6:25–27).

"God is our refuge and strength, a help always near in times of great trouble. That's why we won't be afraid when the world falls apart, when the mountains crumble into the center of the sea, when its waters roar and rage, when the mountains shake because of its surging waves" (Psalm 46:1–3).

"Therefore, stop worrying about tomorrow, because tomorrow will worry about itself. Each day has enough trouble of its own" (Matthew 6:34).

"Ask, and you will receive. Search, and you will find. Knock, and the door will be opened to you. For everyone who asks, receives. Whoever seeks, finds. And to everyone who knocks, the door is opened. Who among you will give your children a stone when they ask for bread? Or give them a snake when they ask for fish? If you who are evil know how to give good gifts to your children, how much more will your heavenly Father give good things to those who ask him" (Matthew 7:7–11).

"I'm not saying this because I need anything, for I have learned how to be content in any circumstance. I know the experience of being in need and of having more than enough; I have learned the secret to being content in any and every circumstance, whether full or hungry or whether having plenty or being poor. I can endure all the things through the power of the one who gives me strength" (Philippians 4:11–13).

"Your way of life should be free from the love of money, and you should be content with what you have. After all, he has said, *I will never leave you or abandon you.* That is why we can confidently say, *The Lord is my helper, and I won't be afraid. What can people do to me?*" (Hebrews 13:5–6).

"A joyful heart brightens one's face, but a troubled heart breaks the spirit" (Proverbs 15–13).

Is your glass half-empty or half-full?

Have you ever overheard two strangers making small talk? Often it is about the weather, politics, or something mutual that they can complain about. Complaining may not be a characteristic that you associate with yourself. However, it doesn't take much to pull one into a conversation, even if he or she is just trying to be nice. Now that sounds like an oxymoron. It's also human nature.

One's work environment is a good example of a place where the glass goes from half full to being half empty quickly. When employees don't have much in common, they will share common criticisms. Negative talk can become toxic and also become habitual.

One word that Gandhi lived by was "ahimsa," which means nonviolence in thought, word, and deed. When it comes to speaking, you probably grew up hearing one of the golden rules: "If you don't have something nice to say, don't say anything at all." I have noticed lately when I am around a certain group of friends there is a lot of cussing mostly out of habit as a way to express themselves. In a sense, cussing is a form of verbal abuse.

Another area that can keep us from being positive is the deeply ingrained judging habit. Charlotte Bell in her book, *Mindful Yoga, Mindful Life,* said "*I saw how nothing in my experience escaped constant evaluation. I even judged my judgments, and judged myself for judging. The feeling that accompanied rampant judging was one of tightness and irritation.*" Become "less judgmental" and more "judge mental". That is, become more aware of this common human tendency to judge others and ourselves.

One of the best ways to have a peaceful and positive life where you always see the glass is as half full is to create an attitude of gratitude. I had a boss and mentor who loved to say, "Sal doesn't see her glass half-full or half-empty. Hers is always overflowing."

On days when you are feeling a little blue—start counting your blessings. It works. Set your intention this week to find gratitude in nothing specific but everything in general.

The following quote by Alice Walker summarizes another way to look at life. "*Look closely at the present you are constructing: it should look like the future you are dreaming.*" This work starts from within a person long before any tangible and significant goals can be accomplished.

- ***Burning Desire (Tapas)***

Burning desire, or Tapas, is your own personal passion for your life's purpose. It is the disciplined use of our energy to better our lives and the lives of others. It is a willingness to do what is necessary to reach the goal. When we generate an attitude of burning passion or enthusiasm toward something, the strength of our convictions generates a momentum that carries us forward. Tapas is a way of directing our energy in order to keep us on track so that we do not waste our time and energy on superficial or trivial matters. When this energy is strong, it is a practice that causes change.

Discovering your dharma—life purpose—is one of the most important steps you can take along our spiritual path. It is the reason for which you were born. When you live your true purpose, you are fully alive, living your fullest potential. If you are not living your dharma, you are merely existing. Per Gandhi, "Be the change you wish to see in the world."

I was blessed to find the road to my life's purpose at an early age. When I was in third grade, I spent a year in bed with rheumatic fever. Family and friends sent postcards from around the world so I could start a collection. It was during this time that I decided I wanted to travel the world when I grew up. It was going to happen by either joining the Peace Corp or by becoming a flight attendant. Even then I felt I was on a journey with God.

During my thirty years in the travel industry, I worked my way up the corporate ladder from flight attendant to president and CEO. I have truly been blessed to have traveled to over 140 countries. In the middle of my career, I began offering "voluntourism" trips where our clients could vacation at a destination while also participating in service work at an orphanage, school, community center, and/or hospital. I eventually obtained my Ph.D. and followed my heart to run the voluntourism operation full-time. I wanted to make a difference in sustainable global projects and a difference in the lives of those who volunteered. Adding yoga in the mix made it even sweeter as retreats could include both the inner and outer journey.

Along the way, I did motivational speeches about "Keys to Success." My first two keys to success were always to find your passion and persevere. That is Tapas... finding your burning desire and doing it.

What's your Dharma? Are you living it? Why not? What are you wanting to be different in your life? How do you make that difference happen?

Here are some exercises to help you find your Dharma:

- Name twenty things that bring you joy. It is in finding your passion that you find your Dharma.

- If there were no rules, and failure was not possible, what would you do?
- Write your own Dharma statement. *My mission in life is to...*

Use the following guidelines:

- Use verbs like heal, produce, teach, manage, inspire...
- Use objects like children, paper products, adults, foreigners...
- Use methods like hospital, family business, English, part-time...
- Include purpose like ministry to families, staying home with children...

Mission Statements:

My mission in life is...
... to help heal children in a hospital setting in order to minister to families.
... to produce paper products in a family business in order to provide for my family.
... to inspire people to travel to developing countries to make a difference in the global community.
... to teach students yoga in order for them to find peace, joy, strength, and flexibility on and off the mat.

- **Jesus's Dharma**

Jesus, himself, worked hard for spiritual growth. Jesus was a human on earth, and besides being the Son of God, his spiritual attainment came through great effort. During his childhood and adolescent years, his initiation from John the Baptist followed by his meditation practices in the wilderness, and his successful struggle over the inner temptations (such as anger, hatred, greed, jealousy, and fear), all took time, perseverance, and patience.

+ **Scripture References on Burning Desire (Tapas)**

"I can endure all these things through the power of the one who gives me strength" (Philippians 4:13).

"Commit your work to the Lord, and your plans will succeed" (Proverbs 16:3).

"So don't throw away your confidence—it brings a great reward. You need to endure so that you can receive the promises after you do God's will" (Hebrews 10:35–36).

"We know that God works all things together for good for the ones who love God, for those who are called according to his purpose" (Romans 8:28).

"Enjoy the Lord, and he will give what your heart asks" (Psalm 37:4).

"Trust in the Lord with all your heart; don't rely on your own intelligence. Know him in all your paths, and he will keep your ways straight" (Proverbs 3:5–6).

"God didn't give us a spirit that is timid but one that is powerful, loving, and self-controlled" (II Timothy 1:7).

Nagging Feeling to Make a Difference: Finding Your Passion

Do you ever get that feeling that life is pretty good but something is missing? You have a great career, family, friends, and outside interests, but you have a nagging feeling that there is something more you should be doing.

It has been an honor and blessing to have met women and men around the world who began with that same little voice within and acted upon it. It has been awe-inspiring to see what these individuals have done to answer their callings.

I first met Natalie, a twenty-seven-year--old Canadian, in Uganda when she was looking for land for a specific project. She ended up building a birthing center and teaching a group of Ugandan women to make jewelry and purses for money. She says, "*The most*

---

empowering thing we can do is to listen to that voice inside, surrender to our path, and collectively make the world a brighter place."

In Cambodia I will never forget my first meeting with Scott Neeson, former president and CEO of Twentieth Century Fox in Hollywood. He asked if I had ever seen extreme poverty. I thought I had, but an hour later, I was standing in one of the world's largest toxic dumps—sixteen acres of it where people lived and worked for pennies a day. Scott obviously felt a major internal shift when he visited the dump in Cambodia while on vacation several years before I had met him. He returned to his job; but after a year, he quit, gave up his houses, boats, and other toys and moved to Phnom Penh. The little voice in his head was telling him to start an orphanage. Beginning with about forty-five orphans, Scott now has more than a thousand children in his many housing and school complexes.

Searching for true abundance took one American woman, Prabha, to India where she lived in a cave on the banks of the Ganges River for many years. Through her quest, she ended up creating a wonderful children's home and school that serves more than 160 children each year. It has been my privilege to journey there every couple years and see her in action.

I keep thinking of the special people who have inspired me to keep listening to that voice inside and the reason I started a center for girls in the heart of the Costa Rican rainforest. My wish for you, dear reader, is to keep listening to your own callings. It may not always be easy, but it is always worth it!

Do What You Cannot Do

Eleanor Roosevelt once said, "Do what you cannot do." If you commit to this statement throughout your life, you will find yourself continually stepping out of your comfort zone and experiencing real personal growth. Courage isn't the absence of fear. Start pursuing new adventures on your "bucket list." Don't have one?

Think of everything you would like to try in your life, write it down, and start checking one item off at a time.

When I was approaching my fortieth birthday, I wanted a challenging new adventure. It took a year to prepare, but I ended up trekking the entire Machu Picchu Trail in Peru, all four mountain passes. It is an incredible feeling when you achieve a goal you have set for yourself. A week after I returned from the trek, it was time to set the next goal. Watching a runner go by, I wondered if I could pursue this activity and added the Indianapolis 500 mini-marathon to my bucket list. A year later I ran my first of seven mini-marathons followed by two full marathons.

A very special friend of mine, Jean Deeds, hiked the entire Appalachian Trail—all 2,180 miles through fourteen states. In her book, *There are Mountains to Climb,* she wrote, "Once you verbalize your intentions and tell the world, you have taken your first step." Her words echoed in my ears when I decided to climb Mt. Kilimanjaro, the highest point in Africa. Around midnight on the fourth evening of the journey, we put on hats with lights and headed up to the summit of 19,341. At 17,500 feet I got full-fledge altitude sickness and only turned back after two other people started down the mountain for the same reason. Being such a goal-oriented person, I didn't even think quitting was an option. Sometimes things are just out of our control. However, there were no regrets. It was an incredible life-changing experience.

Now, every day on the mat, there is always a posture that I would like to conquer. With patience and persistence, it is fun to see what your body and mind can do. There are also times, like Mt. Kilimanjaro, that I let go of something that just doesn't work for me… or my body. As a yoga teacher, I have to admit I can't do a backbend (the wheel or chakrasana in yoga terms), but I've got the "crow" down pat after building up my core strength. (Remember doing tip-ups when you were a kid where you balanced on your hands with your knees resting on the back of your elbows? That's the crow position.) Think you can't do it? Try it now. Do what you think you can't do and surprise yourself.

• *Self-Study (Swadhyaya)*

Self-study, or Swadhyaya, is an inward journey in order to truly learn about ourselves. While it frequently uncovers our strengths, it also relentlessly uncovers our weaknesses and negative tendencies. At these times, it is important to appreciate what we are good at, as well as, to welcome and accept our limitations. It is only through self-study that we can grow and mature as individuals.

There are five obstacles preventing true freedom: ignorance, ego, attachment, aversion/dislike, and fear of death. The best way to deal with these obstacles is to pay attention, acknowledge your feelings, and learn to accept.

Only when individual's look truthfully at who they truly are, change can occur. Yoga brings awareness. It enables us to wake up. See who we are. Then make decisions. Yoga will not tell us how to run our lives. Each of us must deal with our most powerful habitat—our mind.

Personally, this is one of my most important topics of the Yamas and Ni-Yamas, often referred to as the "Ten Commandments of Yoga." I often meditate on these dos and don'ts, committing myself to each. However, until I am truly aware of how I personally interact externally and internally, I cannot make real changes.

+ **Scripture References to Self-Study (Swadhyaya)**

"A time for searching and a time for losing, a time for keeping and a time for throwing away" (Ecclesiastes 3:6).

"Instead, regard Christ as holy in your hearts. Whenever anyone asks you to speak of your hope, be ready to defend it. Yet do this with respectful humility, maintaining a good conscience" (I Peter 3:15–16).

"But anyone who needs wisdom should ask God, whose very nature is to give to everyone without a second thought, without keeping score. Wisdom will certainly be given to those who ask. Whoever asks shouldn't hesitate. They should ask in faith, without doubting.

Whoever doubts is like the surf of the sea, tossed and turned by the wind" (James 1:5–6).

"I turned by mind to know, to investigate, and to seek wisdom, along with an account of things, to know that wickedness is foolishness and folly is madness" (Ecclesiastes 7:25).

"Don't be conformed to the patterns of this world, but be transformed by the renewing of your minds so that you can figure out what God's will is—what is good and pleasing and mature. Because of the grace that God gave me, I can say to each one of you: don't think of yourself more highly than you ought to think. Instead, be reasonable since God has measured out a portion of faith to each one of you" (Romans 12:2–3).

"From now on, brothers and sisters, if anything is excellent and if anything is admirable, focus your thoughts on these things: all that is true, all that is holy, all that is just, all that is pure, all that is lovely, and all that is worthy of praise. Practice these things: whatever you learned, received, heard, or saw in us. The God of peace will be with you" (Philippians 4:8–9).

"Instead, we are God's accomplishment, created in Christ Jesus to do good things. God planned for these good things to be the way that we live our lives" (Ephesians 2:10).

Solitary Moments

When I look back at special moments when traveling, it was those times just being still and taking it all in. Looking down at Machu Picchu in Peru after a five day trek, standing on the Charles Bridge in Prague, watching an Eskimo blanket toss next to the Arctic Ocean in the northern most point of Alaska, doing Tree pose during a yoga class in the heart of the rainforest in Costa Rica... these are the moments that I remember with clarity.

Eagle Creek Park in Indianapolis is one of my most favorite places in the world. Weekly hikes with girlfriends enable us to catch up on each other's lives, be out in nature, and get exercise all at the same time. It also includes stopping somewhere on the trail to take in a specific sight or moment. Recently the stop was next to the water where dozens of egrets were enjoying a swim and turtles were basking on a log. The sky was blue and that feeling of late summer, but not quite fall, felt comforting.

How many times have we told our kids, parents, or even ourselves, "Later?" We have our to-do list that never ends. We often judge our day by what we can check off that list. Wouldn't it be nice to just "be?" Interesting concept. Find time this next week to just *be still.* Take in the wonder and joy for being still and using all your senses.

Eckhart Tolle wrote in his book, *The Power of Now*, that "Glimpses of deep peace are possible whenever a gap occurs in the stream of thought. For most people, such gaps happen rarely and only accidentally, in moments when the mind is rendered "speechless," sometimes triggered by great beauty. Suddenly there is inner stillness."

The present is right now. The present is not the past, and it is not the future. The present is the best gift you can give yourself. A well-known anonymous quote says it all, "Life is not measured by the number of breaths we take, but by the moments that take our breath away." Be still and capture those moments.

• *Surrender to God (Ishvara-Pranidhana)*

Surrender to God, or Ishvara-Pranidhana, is the practice of surrendering to God's will as your own. True freedom comes once you surrender yourself completely to God. Union with God is the real yoga. Maybe if we practiced this ni-yama regularly, all the other disciplines would fall into place.

At the end of most yoga practices, the corpse pose (savasana) is done for at least three minutes or longer. It is accomplished by lying flat on your back with your legs as wide as the mat and the arms a foot away from your hips. Your body should feel a complete surrender into the earth. This particular pose should remind us to let go of anything that no longer serves us in life and leave it on the mat. You have a chance for rebirth and renewal every time you practice yoga.

As a yoga teacher, I often instruct my students that one of the biggest lessons learned on the mat is *letting go*. Let go of expectations and judgments on the mat, then take this principle off the mat. It is a monumental lesson off the mat when one can learn to *let go and let God*.

+ Scripture References to Surrender to God (Ishvara-Pranidhana)

"Faith is the reality of what we hope for, the proof of what we don't see" (Hebrews 11:1).

"Don't chase after what you will eat and what you will drink. Stop worrying. All the nations of the world long for these things. Your Father knows that you need them. Instead, desire his kingdom and these things will be given to you as well" (Luke 12:29–30).

"Trust in the Lord forever, for the Lord is a rock for all ages" (Isaiah 26:4).

"But the fruit of the Spirit is love, joy, peace, patience, kindness, goodness, faithfulness, gentleness, and self-control" (Galatians 5:22).

"Peace I leave with you. My peace I give you. I give to you not as the world gives. Don't be troubled or afraid" (John 14:27).

"The people who love your instruction enjoy peace—and lots of it. There's no stumbling for them! Lord, I wait for your saving help. I do what you've commanded. I keep your laws; I love them so much!" (Psalm 119:165–167).

All of the disciplines employed in the practice of yoga are necessary to promote physical and mental health. By focusing on the *Yamas* and *Ni-Yamas*, individuals gain an atmosphere of peace and serenity and a profound understanding of themselves, within, as well as, in the outside world. Yoga is a spiritual discipline allowing individuals to transcend from a human realm to a oneness with God.

Exercises:

1. List four of your strengths.
2. Describe what you are doing when you are most comfortable?
3. What is your Dharma? (Note: This is not necessarily your job)
4. Do a vision board of what you want in your future? Cut words and pictures from magazines and paste to a large poster board.
5. I feel most like me when I _____.
6. What I like most about myself is _____.
7. What I most value in my life right now is _____.
8. Right now in life I am _____. This year I would like to _____.
9. Write your eulogy. Example: "Here lies Sally Bassett. She lived a full life experiencing all four corners of the world, raised two incredible daughters… and lived her life guided by God.
10. Write a dialogue between you and your Guardian Angel. What advice would your Guardian Angel give you?
11. I have a dream to _____but _____. How do you change the "but?"
12. Identify three additional scriptures for each *Ni-Yamas*.

Letting Go

Do you have a child that is going off to college for the first time... or even starting kindergarten? Are you trying to get over an unhealthy relationship? Is grieving for someone or something not letting you move on? What would *you* like to let go of in your life?

As parents when we raise our children, we strive to give them "roots to grow and wings to fly." Sometimes, however, it is harder than we think to truly let go for our sake more than theirs. Letting go of anything that is holding us back from being content or truly happy is something that we all have to purposefully do. It does not mean we care less. Instead, it is the realization that nothing is permanently ours in the first place.

When I was single, I remember having an unhealthy crush on one of our pilots. At a weekend retreat there was an activity where I sat across from an empty chair and told the person why the relationship wasn't healthy. Gradually the chair was moved back a couple of feet at a time visualizing that person leaving my life. The exercise worked because I confronted that I needed to let go of a bad situation and move toward the future with joy.

One of the biggest lessons I learn on the yoga mat is learning to let go of expectations and judgment. When we learn to let go of the small stuff, we can then learn to let go of the bigger concerns in life.

In the ancient book of the *Bhagavad Gita,* it is filled with lessons about letting go, including the following passage:

> *"Though the unwise cling to their actions, watching for results, the wise are free of attachments, and act for the well-being of the whole world."*

A lotus pond is a great analogy of how beautiful letting go and rising above it all can be. The lotus flower starts out as a seed, rises from the lowest point in muddy water and grows upward toward the light. Once it rises up, it never touches the murky water again and is one of the most extraordinary and revered flowers in the world.

May you commit to letting go of something that is not working in your life right now. Letting go often means rising above it all to blossom like never before.

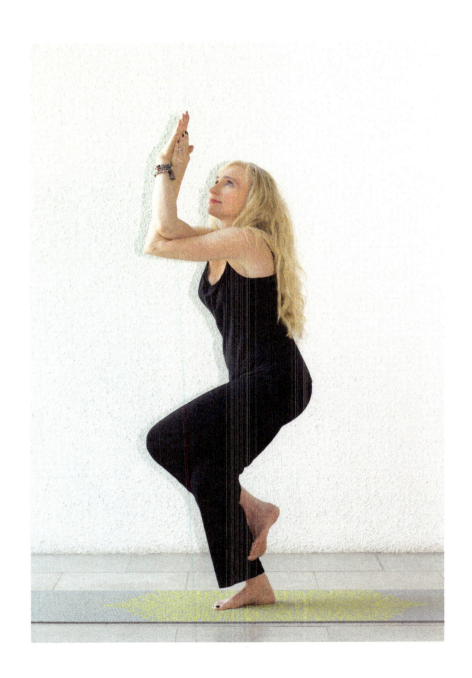

CHAPTER 4

The Third Limb of Yoga: Postures or Asanas

Asanas, the body postures and poses associated with yoga, constitute the third limb of yoga. Most people begin a yoga practice to embrace the physical benefits yoga provides. They also discover yoga's power to reduce stress, nurture mindfulness, and improve overall heath. But the underlying purpose of practicing asanas is to eventually prepare the body for sitting in prayer and meditation for an extended period of time. It is in disciplining the body one can maintain the correct posture for meditation without fatique or physical and mental restlessness.

There are many benefits of the asanas including *improved balance, strength, flexibility, endurance, and reduction of stress and anxiety.* Chronic health conditions can also be addressed and, in some cases, cured.

There are hundreds of yoga poses that also include many variations or modifications that can be used according to the ability of the person. The poses are known by both their English and Sanskrit names. Some poses include: mountain pose (tadasana), plow (halasana), fish (matsyasana), boat (navasana), and corpse (savasana).

Throughout the poses, the body should always be steady and comfortable. This is contradictory to the popular "no pain, no gain" philosophy. Each pose focuses on strengthening and balancing different parts of the body. As a person moves, or flows, from one pose to another, the muscles work together to move the body in different directions thus increasing the overall physical benefits than each pose individually can accomplish.

Every move is done in conjunction with breath – an inhale or exhale. The intentionality of breathing into and through each movement is a key factor for getting into, remaining in, and moving out of a pose. This focus on the breath is instrumental in maintaining mindfulness of being in the moment and is essential to prevent soreness. (More on breath follows in the next chapter)

Historically, yoga poses evolved from the need to create a healthy body in order to move more readily to the state of meditation. When the body is filled with stress and tension, it is hard for the mind to be calm. The physical freedom achieved from the postures increases the ability to sit in meditative silence. Yoga, therefore, contributes to spiritual growth and improves the quality of life. While the practicing of the asanas is only one step in achieving peace through yoga, they are a key step in preparing the physical body for the remaining limbs.

When doing an asana practice, remember the body is a considered a sacred vehicle. Listen to it. Remember, there is no comparison or competition in yoga. It is an individual practice that encourages you to find your "edge" (the furtheset point of a stretch that can be made without pain) in a pose and explore it. Sometimes resistance is a path of learning. Asana practice is not just about getting toned, but it includes cultivating an open mind and heart. Challenging asanas teach you to breathe, relax, let go of your ego, and to release judgement or criticism. Yoga is about finding empowerment as well as humility. There is a limit to flexibility and contorting your body should not be the goal. The rest is all ego.

What does mountain pose or any of the postures (asanas) have to do with uniting with God? By going within and being aware of the body, you come into the "now". Sometimes I must remind myself that it isn't about stillness of the mind as much as it is being mindful. We can go from point A to point B in a car and never remember getting there. In this regard, washing dishes can be a form of yoga. Truly being mindful on the mat sounds so simple, but most people tend to be thinking about the past or the future versus being totally present. We are not our thoughts! Being mindful during our yoga time allows us to rediscover who we really are.

Evolution of physical fitness is mental fitness. Mental stress can precede a physical disease. Therefore, by focusing our minds while moving through asanas, a person is able to eliminate those psychosomatic issues and address those legitimate ones.

As an adjunct professor at Butler University, I teach yoga to students for college credit. Many of my students sign up for the class to reduce stress. Stress has been linked to the six leading causes of death in our society: heart disease, cancer, lung ailments, cirrhosis of the liver, suicide and accidents. Stress shows up in the body before the mind even knows it is there. Stress is not simply what is happening to a person as much as it is how that person perceives and deals with the effects of stress on his or her being.

Scripture reminds us of the importance of caring for our bodies. The Apostle Paul wrote in II Corinthians 6:16, "We are the temple of the living God" and in I Corinthians. 6:20, "Honor God with your body." Yoga is a way to help us fully inhabit our bodies and to begin using them to more fully actualize what God calls us to be. To carry the life of God in our bodies is both a gift and a responsibility.

I like to remind my students that they will reach the point that their practice is their life and their life is their practice.

Through asana practice, our bodies become more flexible and youthful. Some poses are similar to what we did as children like the wheel (backbend), headstand, or tree while others bring us into new body positions, such as warrior, pigeon, and crow. As our bodies become stronger and more flexible, we can indeed follow Jesus' admonition that we enter the Kingdom of God as a child. And, when the energy of the Holy Spirit is in us, we are truly alive, enabling us to understand the sufferings of others and become motivated to help transform our world. This empathetic worldview ties us all to others spiritually. Thus, in a very real sense, yoga can become a spiritual practice.

Worship through yoga also deepens our relationship with God. At the start of a yoga practice, the individual sets an intention. These can be selecting one of the Yamas and/or Niyamas to focus on, identifying a particular goal for that session, or dedicating the practice to someone or something. Yoga practice can even be a form of a silent prayer. It is for me.

Sometimes words alone cannot express the thanksgiving we feel toward God. "Sun Salutations" (a series of flowing poses) can be a form of worship much like a liturgical dance. Sun Salutations begin by lifting our hands up to heaven in praise then bowing down, humbling ourselves before God.

+ Scripture References for Posture (Asanas)

"Or don't you know that your body is a temple of the Holy Spirit who is in you? Don't you know that you have the Holy Spirit from God, and you don't belong to yourselves?" (I Corinthians 6:19).

"So, brothers and sisters, because of God's mercies, I encourage you to present your bodies as a living sacrifice that is holy and pleasing to God." (Romans 12:1).

"So then let's also run the race that is laid out in front of us, since we have such a great cloud of witnesses surrounding us. Let's throw off any extra baggage, get rid of the sin that trips us up, and fix our eyes on Jesus, faith's pioneer and perfecter. He endured the cross, ignoring the shame, for the sake of the joy that was laid out in front of him, and sat down at the right side of God's throne." (Hebrews 12: 1-2).

"While physical training has some value, training in holy living is useful for everything. It has promise for this life and the life to come." (I Timothy 4:8).

"The eye is the lamp of the body. Therefore, if your eye is healthy, your whole body will be full of light. But if your eye is bad, your whole body will be full of darkness. If then the light in you is darkness, how terrible that darkness will be!" (Matthew 6:22-23).

"It's a physical body when it's put into the ground, but it's raised as a spiritual body. If there's a physical body, there's also a spiritual body. So it is also written, *The first human, Adam, became a living person,* and the last Adam became a spirit that gives life. But the physical body comes first, not the spiritual one—the spiritual body comes afterward. The first human was from the earth made from dust; the second human is from heaven. The nature of the person made of dust is shared by people who are made of dust, and the nature of the heavenly person is shared by heavenly people. We will look like the heavenly person in the same way as we have looked like the person made from dust." (I Corinthians 15: 44-49).

Asana Template for *Yoga through Christ*

Throughout the practice: *Lift up your face, arms, and heart to give praise and bow down humbly to give gratitude*

Seated Pose

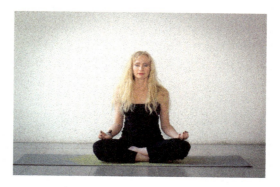

- Set the intention of the practice by choosing one Yama or Niyama along with a correlating passage(s) from the Bible. Reflect on this intention and how it resonates in your life. Say a prayer for the practice.

Poses on back

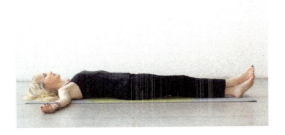

- ***Corpse Pose*** – Start by laying on your back with your ankles crossed and your arms straight out to the side (like Jesus on the cross). Corpse pose allows us to let everything go that no longer serves us.
- ***Windshield Wipers*** - Place the soles of the feet on the earth as wide as the mat. Drop the knees to one side then continue moving them back and forth like windshield wipers with your head turning the opposite direction of the knees. (Inhale as the knees move, exhale as they find stillness)

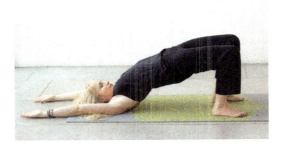

- ***Bridge Pose*** - Place the soles of the feet on the mat hips distance apart and close to the sit bones. Slowly lift the hips in the air while bringing the arms over your head, then slowly roll down one vertebrae at a time along with the arms at the same pace. Continue this flow six or seven times. (Inhale as you lift up, exhale as you come back down)

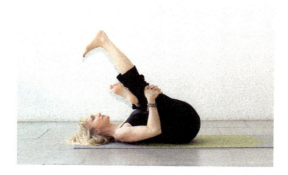

- *Modified Pigeon* - Place the right ankle on the top of the left thigh (like sitting man-style in a chair), bring your hands behind the left thigh. Gently draw your left leg toward your upper torso and hold for several breaths. Now reverse, placing the left ankle on the top of the right thigh.

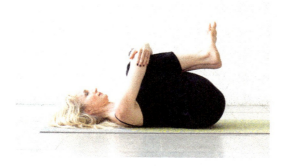

- *Spine Massage* - Bring knees into the chest and rock left to right massaging the lower part of the back.

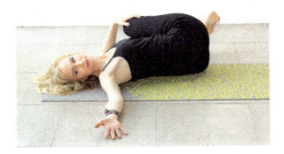

- ***Spinal Twist*** – Place arms out like a "T." Drop the knees to the right, take the right hand on top of the left thigh, lift the head, and look to the left. Take four to six full deep breaths. Reverse sides.

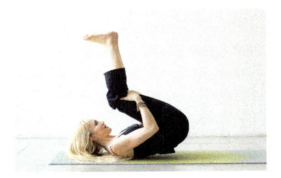

- ***Upward Roll*** – With clasped hands behind bent knees, rock and roll front to back on your spine three to five times before coming up to a comfortable seated position.

Seated Poses

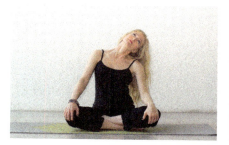
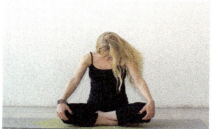

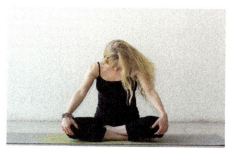

-   *Neck Circles* - Sit with back straight, chin toward chest, pretend you have paint on your nose to make a big circle and slowly begin rolling your head right on the inhale and exhaling as ear comes to the other side; complete approximately five on each side with eyes closed.

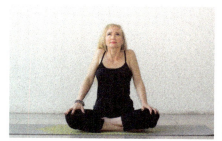
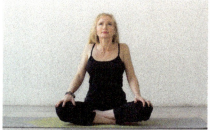

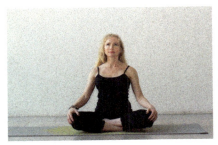 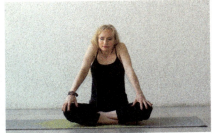

- ***Shoulder Rolls*** – With eyes closed, slowly inhale and roll shoulders up and then exhale as you roll them back and down; complete approximately six times with the intention of letting all thoughts and concerns roll off your shoulders.

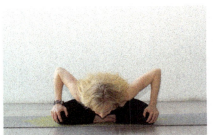 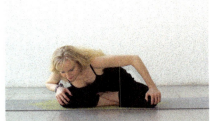

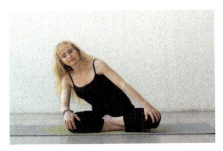 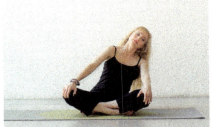

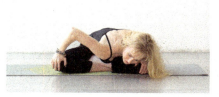 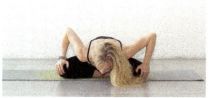

- ***Torso/Body Circles*** - Place palms face down on knees, nose toward the earth, inhale as you circle your entire upper torso to the right and exhale as you come circle to the left. Eyes are closed as you complete five rotations, then switch out legs (reversing the leg that is in front) and repeat by going in the other direction. This pose is meditation in motion.

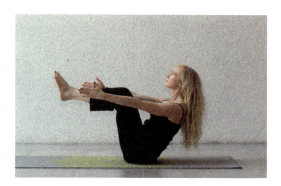

- ***Boat Pose*** - Roll back off your sit-bones slightly, bring both feet off the ground and find yourself in a V shape, knees can be bent slightly, back straight. Breathe deeply for approximately five counts.

Poses on Knees

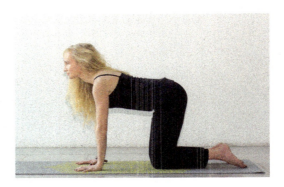

- *Table* – Roll onto your hands and knees. Hands are directly under hips and back is neutral (flat).

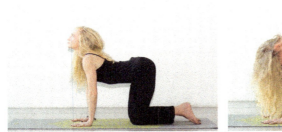 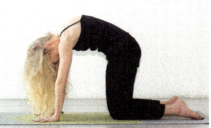

- *Cat/Cow* – From Table, drop your belly while lifting your chest/heart and head causing an arch in your back going into Cow pose. Next drop your chin to your chest, while pushing your belly button up towards your spine, and creating a "hump" with your spine thus forming the Cat pose. Inhale into Cow and exhale into Cat. Repeat eight to ten times.

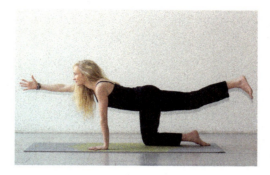

- ***Star Burst*** – Reach right arm and left leg out to be parallel to the floor. Hold for several breaths then add crunches with opposite elbow to opposite knee. Return to Table position and reverse sides, extending left arm and right leg and complete the series.

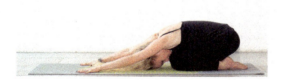

- ***Child's Pose*** – From Table, push hips back towards heels. Drop chest towards the earth, extend arms forward beside ears with palms facing down. This is a relaxing pose representing innocence transformed. "Let all the little children come to me."

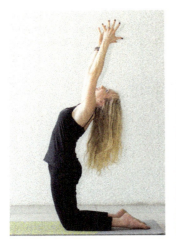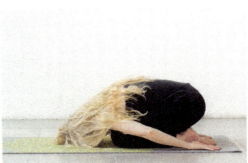

- ***Praise & Gratitude*** – With a flowing movement, rise up on your knees, reach arms up and back, lifting your heart and arms to the heavens and return to child's pose. Repeat approximately six times. This symbolizes lifting the heart in praise and bowing down in gratitude and humility.

Standing Poses

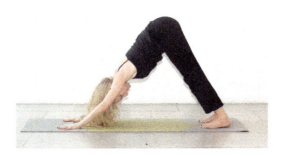

- ***Downward Facing Dog*** – Return to Table then lift your hips towards the ceiling, pushing into your heels and palms.

(Pause in this position to feel the pyramid of this pose representing Father, Son, Holy Ghost)

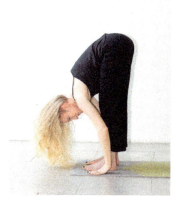

- ***Standing Forward Fold*** – From Downward Facing Dog, walk your feet toward your hands, bending your knees along the way. Hold on to opposite elbows with your hands and hang. Relax your head and let gravity do the work as you take five to seven long deep breaths. Slowly roll yourself up into a standing pose.

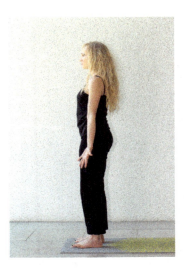

- *Mountain Pose* – Feet are hip width apart, shoulders roll up and back, chin is parallel to the ground, tailbone is tucked under, arms are at the side with palms facing forward. Your legs are engaged by grounding down into the earth from which we were made and where we find strength.
- *Sun Salutations C* – one to two times (Refer to diagram)

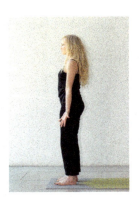 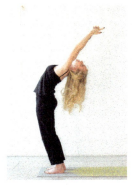 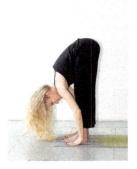

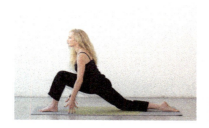
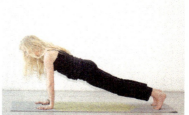

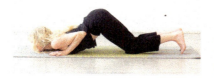
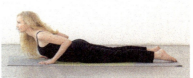

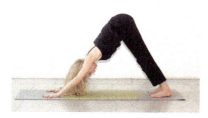
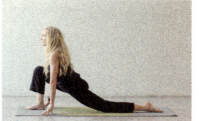

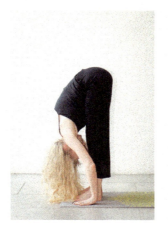
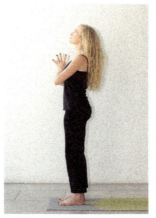

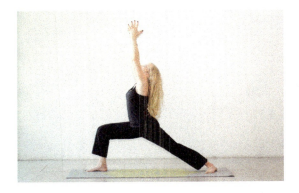

- *Warrior I* – Bring the right foot to the front of the mat and place the left foot at the back of the mat at a 45 degree angle. Bend the right knee over the ankle so only the big toe can be seen. Place hands on your hips and rotate left hip forward to be parallel to the front of the mat. Lift your hands to the heavens, close your eyes and make a prayer request.

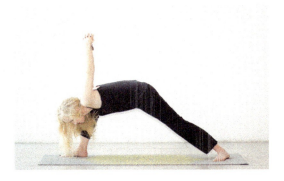

- *Humble Warrior* – Bring your arms around to your back, linking the fingers together. Bow down with arms reaching back and know God heard your prayers.

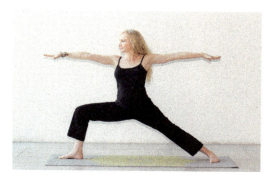

- *Warrior II* – From Warrior I open your body out to the left with arms reaching parallel to the earth. Adjust so the front heel aligns with the arch of the back foot. Focus on the left middle finger and commit to staying the course with your prayers.

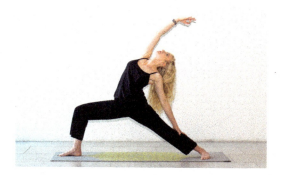

- *Exalted Warrior* - Maintain Warrior II, drop the back arm and place against thigh, rotate the front palm towards the ceiling, bringing the arm up and reaching back. Toss back anything that you need to *let go* and *let God*.

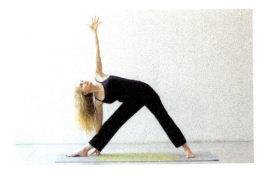

- *Triangle* - Return to Warrior II. Straighten the front leg, extend the front arm forward until it can reach no further, then pivot the arms placing the bottom hand against the leg with the opposite arm reaching towards the ceiling. This pose represents the Trinity.

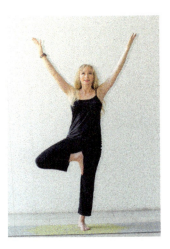

- *Tree Pose* - Ground down in your left foot and place the right foot above the ankle, on the calf, or on the thigh. (Never place the foot on the knee). Raise arms above head in a "V" formation. Symbolically, this represents the grounding of your faith and the sending of blessings out into the world.

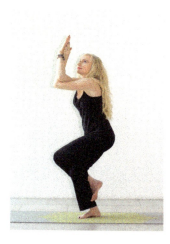

- *Eagle* – Bend your knees and cross your left leg over right. Tuck your left foot behind your right calf, if you can. Wrap your left arm under your right arm and bring thumbs to face you. This pose represents taking flight and having faith. Repeat the standing poses on other side.

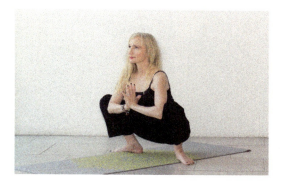

- *Yogi Squat* - Move heels to the edge of the mat with toes off the mat. Reach arms up and move hands into prayer pose while slowly lowering your body down to a squat. Press the elbows into the thighs and lift the heart. Take a minimum of five breaths.

Seated Poses

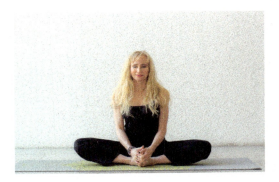

- ***Cobbler's Pose*** - Place both soles of the feet together, hold on to the toes, and bring the heels toward the body. Folding forward is an option.

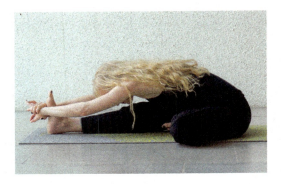

- ***Head to Knee Pose*** – Extend legs straight out on mat. Place one foot along the side of the opposite inner thigh and fold forward. Repeat on the other side.
- ***Easy Pose*** – Cross your legs in a seated position with back straight.

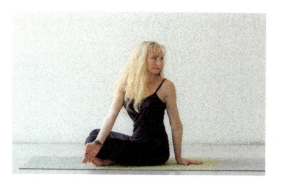

- ***Spinal Twist*** - In Easy Pose take your left hand to the opposite knee and windmill the right hand up and around close to the back. Breathe into the twist. Switch sides.

"*Practice becomes firmly grounded when well attended to for a long time, without break and in all earnestness.*" Yoga Sutra 1:14. Yoga practice requires these three qualities: patience, devotion and faith. Without discipline nothing can be achieved.

Additional Poses for Your Practice

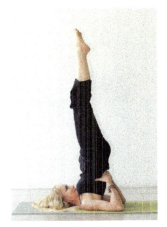

Shoulder Stand

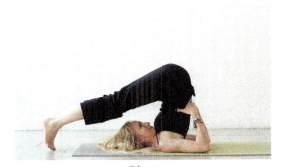

Plow

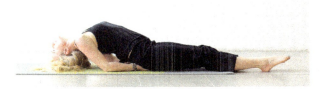

Fish

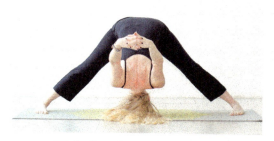

Wide Standing Forward Fold

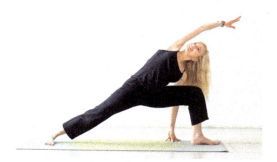

Side Angle Stretch

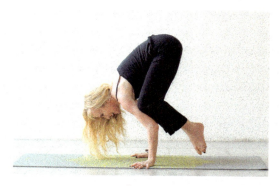

Crow

****

Exercise:

1. Discribe how your body image affected you throughout your life? How can you let all judgment go regarding your physical practice?
2. If you are a certified yoga teacher offer the practice to five friends or family members.
3. What would you like to lift up and ask God in Warrior I?
4. What would you like to focus on in the future in Warrior II?
5. What would you like to "let go" of to become an "exalted" warrior? Circle one: pride, anger, greed, impatience, hatred, jealousy, selfishness, other_____.
6. What would you like *more* of to become a stronger spiritual/bhakti warrior? Circle one: strength, courage, balance, grace, truth, wisdom, love, other_____.

****

Issues Live in our Tissues

If you have something unresolved in your life, it often creates toxins that can be manifested in many ways. Is something covering some past drama that is causing an addictive type personality? Addictions do not necessarily have to be just alcohol and drugs. Addictions can range from uncontrolled eating, shopping, gambling, hoarding, smoking, sex, working, and other human activities in excess. These things can be a way to cope with life's stresses. Anything that takes someone out of the present moment can turn into an addiction.

A yoga colleague and friend of mine, Nikki Myers, developed a program called the *Yoga of 12-Step Recovery* (Y12SR). Her program helps individuals with all types of addictions by using discussion, yoga, breath work and meditation to explore addiction and recovery within the mind/body continuum. It weaves together the wisdom of yoga and the practical tools of 12-step programs.

Yoga helps individuals find the balance and complete integration to release physical stress, emotional pain, and prevent *dis-ease*. First, yoga helps individuals ground themselves so they can turn their lives around and set sail on their own spiritual voyages. On the mat, yoga teaches: "How we do *anything* is how we do *everything*."

When you clear out the issues that are living in your tissues, you will start feeling connected and grateful to the world around you. You will be restored and renewed. Instead of running away from emotions, breathe in the negative feeling, and then breathe out the opposite emotion. For example, if you are dealing with anger, breathe out peace.

You Are What You Eat, Do and Think

Wherever I got separated from my mom, as a child, I would just have to listen for her laughter to to tell me where she was. My mother has always loved laughter. However, there were always two things she didn't like to do: exercise and eat healthy, green food.

Now at 85, my mom still loves to laugh, and she still dreads walking more than a few feet (unless it is shopping) and asks the same questions every minute or so. She has dementia. I can't help wonder if she would have more of a quality of life today if she would have cared more about her health.

James H. West wrote, *"Health is a large word. It embraces not the body only, but the mind and spirit as well;…and not today's pain or pleasure alone, but the whole being and outlook of a man."*

What if, just what if, our bodies are the temple of our souls? Would you do anything different? Let's consider the following ideas:

* ***You are what you Eat***

You already know what the implications are with obesity. If over eating is a challenge, start with cutting down portion sizes and drink a full glass of water prior to every meal. Try to make a difference in yout friends' and your family's eating habits as well.

Simple decisions like packing healthier lunches for your kids, and bringing good options to those family get-togethers and workplace pitch-ins can send a positive message about the importance of choosing healthy food.

- **You are what you DO (or don't do):**

Most Americans are sitting 4 hours a day in front of a computer. At the end of a long day, try not to be a couch potato. Don't ask, "What should I do or not do?" Do something! Get your endorphins going and create energy in your body that you forgot you had.

- **You are what you THINK:**

According to the Laboratory of Neuro Imaging, the average person has about 70,000 thoughts a day. If those thoughts are stressful, you literally can subtract years from your life. Here's a question for you: If you didn't know how old you were, what would you be? Our natural God-given state is meant to be peace and joy. May you seek those two things with your whole heart.

From <u>Go In and In: Poems from the Heart of Yoga</u> by Donna Faulds.

YOGA

Yoga is not about the pose.
It's not the alignment of
toes or hips or shoulders.
It's not about the form.

Yoga is an invitation to
explore, not a command
performance. It speaks
the language of the soul.

In the flow of breath and
motion, yoga coaxes us
from the confines of the
known, across the silent
threshold into vastness.

Yoga is the union of prayer
and movement, guided from
inside. It is healing and the
joy of saying yes to life.

Breathe, relax and feel the
body receive its own truth.
The seed of freedom flowers
within each of us whenever
we are open to what's real.

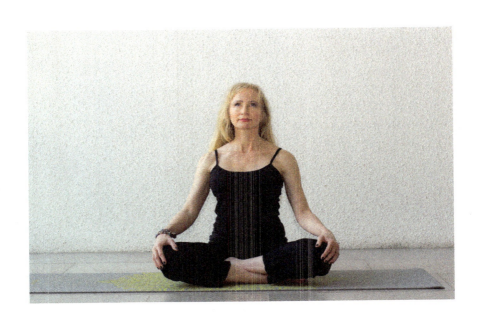

CHAPTER 5

The Fourth Limb of Yoga: Breath Control or Pranayama

Pranayama, the fourth limb of yoga, is the formal practice of controlling the breath or mindful breathing. This Sanskrit word comes from "prana," meaning life-force and "ayama" which means to draw out. As the parts of the word suggest, *pranayama* is an extension of the breath. Through the practice of pranayama, people can learn to change and control the rate, quality, and pattern of the breath. We use so little of our lung capacity. Studies have shown as little as 20 percent of our lungs are used while we are watching television. Expanding our lung capacity creates energy as well as calmness, an oxymoron at its best.

Pranayama allows the body to operate more efficiently. Through the regulation of the breath, an individual can begin taking steps to become healthier. While breathing normally, the average person only uses about half of the lungs' capacity. While practicing pranayama, up to eighty percent of the lungs' capacity is used. The body then has access to more oxygen, and red blood cells can carry that oxygen to the rest of the body at almost a maximum efficiency. Immediately, the entire body benefits and can function better. The body can then heal itself quickly and more efficiently.

In order to effectively improve breathing, it is important to regulate all parts of the breathing process. First, breathing through the nose is most effective when trying to regulate the breath. By taking in air through the nose, it is filtered, warmed, and moistened. This is the ideal condition for air arriving in the lungs, as opposed to air that is taken in through the mouth.

The practice of pranayama massages the internal organs and rids the body of toxins when the exhalation is longer than the inhalation. When breathing normally, a person will usually only fill and empty the top and middle thirds of the lungs. It is important to fill and empty the bottom third of the lungs as well by contracting the stomach up and back. We call that the three-part breath.

Of course, breathing is necessary to keep humans alive, as the body requires oxygen in order to survive, but using breathing techniques can positively affect a person's thoughts and actions as well. A happy or content person breathes more naturally and rhytmic, and the body is mostly at rest. In order to eliminate stress, a change in breathing pattern can be extremely beneficial. Breathing rhythmically is important in self-healing, since stress often causes breathing to be irregular and restricted. Pranayama can help to heal the body by regulating the breath.

Actually, the most physical healing part of yoga is pranayama not the asanas. Are your asanas following your breath, or is your breath following asanas? Breathe as if you truly believe each breath would enrich your health. It will.

Pranayama is also useful to help clear the mind of any concerns and troubles. By focusing on the breath, it is easier to eliminate excess thoughts. This emptying of the mind is important for meditation. In order to truly benefit from the study of yoga, one needs to put all of the eight limbs of yoga together. Only through self-restraints, individual practices, postures, breath control, sense withdrawal, concentration, and meditation, will a person find profound, absorbed meditation, and oneness with God.

Breathe, believe, and you will receive. Pranayama is the bridge between the physical and the spiritual. Space is generated, and your spiritual self has a place to live.

A Few Types of Pranayama

Focus on the breath. We use so little of our lung capacity so not only will focusing on breath be a meditation, but it will also bring both calmness and energy.

- Three Part Breath: calming and cleansing
  Fill the lower part of your lungs, middle part, then all the way to the top of the lungs. Exhale slowly top, middle, bottom—contracting your stomach muscles to get all stale air and toxins out of your body. Continue filling the lungs like you are filling a pitcher of water from bottom to top then empty top to bottom.

- Victorious Breath (*Ujjayi*): heating and cleansing
  Open your mouth to get a feel of how the breath should sound and exhale like you are trying to fog up a window. Now close your mouth; practice the *ujayii* breath with the sound/restriction at the back of your throat being louder than your thoughts.

- Alternating Nostril Breathing (*Anuloma Viloma*): balancing and calming
  Place your middle and pointer finger on your forehead. Cover your left nostril with your ring finger and inhale completely through the right nostril; cover the right nostril with your thumb and release the ring finger; exhale through the left nostril. Inhale through the same nostril; cover and release the other nostril as you exhale. Continue for several minutes.

- Breath of Fire (*Kapalabhati*): cleansing and purifying
  To get a sense of how this breath work should feel physically, stick out your tongue and pant like a dog for a moment. Now close your mouth and feel the same sensation in your belly as you exhale rapidly. Your focus is on the exhale rather than the inhale. Do as many as 27 rapid exhales if you can.

- Bellows Breath (*Bhastrika*): energizing and cleansing

Raise your arms up toward where the ceiling meets the wall. Exhale powerfully by bringing your elbows into the sides of your body and hands into fists. Do this ten to 15 times maximum at a rapid speed.

- Ego Eradicator: energizing and cleansing both physical and spiritually

Raise your hands up over your head in a V-shape with only your thumbs raised to the heavens and other fingers tucked in. Close your eyes and do 27 to 54 Breath of Fires focusing on the exhale. This repetition allows you to get rid of anything the ego is holding back so that you can go to the higher levels in yoga.

Note: 108 is an auspicious number in yoga, the same as number of beads on a mala necklace. 108 Sun Salutations are often done at the change of seasons. The number can also be broken down to 54 when practicing certain yoga postures or breathing exercises; or breakdown even further to 27.

+ **Scripture References on Breath (Pranayama)**

"The Lord God formed the human from the topsoil of the fertile land and blew life's breath into his nostrils. The human came to life" (Genesis 2: 7).

"God's spirit made me; the Almighty's breath enlivens me" (Job 33:4).

"In whose grasp is the life of everything, the breath of every person?" (Job 12:10).

"Nor is God served by human hands, as though he needed something, since he is the one who gives life, breath, and everything else" (Acts 17:25).

"Let every living thing praise the Lord" (Psalm 150:6).

"God the Lord says—the one who created the heavens, the one who stretched them out, the one who spread out the earth and its offspring, the one who gave breath to its people and life to those who walk on it" (Isaiah 42:5).

"But after three and a half days, the breath of life from God entered them, and they stood on their feet. Great fear came over those who saw them. Then they heard a loud voice from heaven say to them, 'Come up here.' And they went up to heaven in a cloud, while their enemies watched them" (Revelation 11:11–12).

Exercise:

- Practice two types of *pranayama* every day for three to five minutes for a week and begin the path toward meditation.

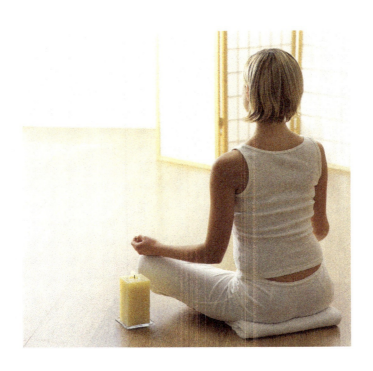

CHAPTER 6

The Fifth Limb of Yoga – Sense Withdrawal or Pratyahara

The remaining four limbs of yoga are all related to deepening our capacity to meditate. Scripture is filled with an abundance of references related to prayer and meditation. Yoga provides a step-by-step method for developing a strong and vibrant meditative life. The first four limbs enable us to physically be ready to meditate. Medition then starts with the fifth limb of yoga, which is withdrawing from the senses, or pratyahara. This is defined in Sanskrit as "gaining mastery over external influences." By withdrawing from the senses, an individual can turn inward. Even withdrawing from just one or two of the five senses (hearing, feeling, tasting, smelling, and seeing) will enable a person to go inward and become detached from the physical world.

Pratyahara practices lead to a profound state of relaxation and expanded self-awareness. The problem arises when we can't let go of sensations. There are a variety of ways to build this practice. These include going to bed on time and or getting at least eight hours of sleep, so the body is physically rested and ready to concentrate. Occasionally refrain from food, talking, any physical activity, and/or entertainment to help foster relaxation. By actively restraining the senses and focusing the mind in guided relaxation practices and meditation, you create habits that support more mindfulness and inner peace. Turn off the television, close your eyes, focus on the silence. See what happens.

As a person progresses through these steps of withdrawal, the state of pratyahara is reached with greater ease. Sounds are still registered, but they do not cause a disturbance in the person. Simply put, people in pratyahara are in the world but not of it. The practice of pratyahara is like returning to your true self.

An Invitation for the Holy Spirit to Enter

Once withdrawn from the senses individuals go deeper into their being, and the Holy Spirit can now respond to the invitation to enter in and accomplish the work of God in us. The Holy Ghost is the sacred, invisible vibratory power of God. It brings God's power to life. *On occasion, you may actually experience a spiritual ecstasy that vibrates throughout your entire body.*

As we descend to the center of our own nothingness, it is then possible for the Spirit to lead us to find God. One can experience the joy of being filled with the Holy Spirit. Withdrawing from the senses will eventually reveal the light of the spiritual eye.

Pratyahara Exercises:

Purposely practice withdrawing from one sense at a time. Here are some examples that also improve mindfulness.

1. Go into a completely dark room or closet. See what senses are heightened when you are not using the sense of sight. I recently did this in my cabin bathroom while on a cruise ship. It was pitch black and I became instantly aware of the movement of the ship for the first time. The light sounds of suds popping in the sink after doing some laundry were a delight.

2. Close sound out by going under water or covering your ears with your index fingers. One of my joys in life is swimming under water or even floating on top where all sounds are diminished. By closing the eyes, one gains a higher degree of awareness. One afternoon in Belize I will never forget diving into the water and floated up from the ocean floor on my back looking through goggles. The water on top sparkled from the sun, the sky was a beautiful blue, and my body felt light and free.

3. Get three or four different bite size pieces of foods that you can smell, explore, and simply chew slowly to savor the taste and texture. Do the chewing with your eyes closed to enhance the sense of taste. This exercise has been fun to do with my students on retreats as we taste things like pineapple, chocolate, coconut, a nut, and other seasonal produce. You will be surprised that you will feel more satisfied than if you had just eaten a five-course meal.

+ **Scripture References for Withdrawing from the Senses (Pratyahara)**

"God doesn't look at things like humans do. Humans see only what is visible to the eyes, but the Lord sees into the heart" (1 Samuel 16:7b).

"Don't be conformed to the patterns of this world, but be transformed by the renewing of your mind so that you can figure out what God's will is—what is good and pleasing and mature" (Romans 12: 2).

"Wine is a mocker; beer a carouser. Those it leads astray won't become wise" (Proverbs 20:1).

"Pray like this: Our Father who is in heaven, uphold the holiness of your name. Bring in your kingdom so that your will is done on earth as it's done in heaven. Give us the bread we need for today. Forgive us for the ways we have wronged you, just as we also forgive those who have wronged us. And don't lead us into temptation but rescue us from the evil one" (Matthew 6:9–13).

Exercises:
- Give two examples of how you could practice pratyahara off the mat by withdrawing from certain senses.
- "Prune" back anything in your life that is stopping you from having quiet time to worship and practice yoga. Make the time. Examine your priorities. Are you involved in so many activities that you are ineffective? Are these activities, meetings, or obligations bringing joy and fulfillment? God doesn't want you to always do more FOR Him. He wants you to be more WITH Him.

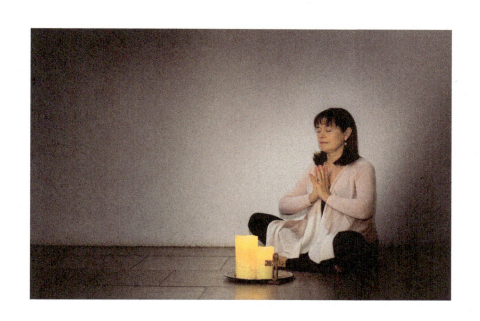

CHAPTER 7

The Sixth Limb of Yoga: Concentration or Dharana Prayer/Talking to God

Concentration, or dharana, is the sixth of the Eight Limbs of Yoga. It builds upon the fifth limb of yoga, pratyahara, which is withdrawing from the senses and allows the Holy Spirit to fill you. Dharana draws the senses to a singular object or focus—Jesus. The mind concentrates without wavering and avoids all other thoughts.

The goal of concentration and meditation, is to attain a connection with Jesus. For successful concentration to occur, a person must have a good understanding of the previous five limbs of yoga. Worry and grief, which should be eliminated in the second limb of yoga, are considered to be two of the biggest obstacles to a person's ability to concentrate.

Other suggestions to help build concentration skills that will enable one to go inward are to focus on a lit candle for five to ten minutes, or to become totally absorbed in the movement of an insect or activity of an ant hill, to so mindfully wash your car that you are aware of each movement you make.

• *Praying to Jesus*

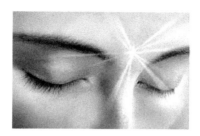

To begin, take your inner attention to your sixth chakra, Ajna Chakra or your third eye—our "spiritual eye". This is located right between your eyebrows at the front of your brain. There you will find Jesus. Seeking Jesus' face for enjoyment, not just his hands for blessings, can unfold an awesome spiritual experience for the practioner of dharana.

Paramahansa Yogananda's words have been a confirmation for what I have personally experienced. "By the right method of meditation and devotion, with the eyes closed and concentrated on the spiritual eye, the devotee knocks at the gates of heaven. When the eyes are focused and still, and the breath and mind are calm, a light begins to form in the forehead. Eventually, with deep concentration, the tricolored light of the spiritual eye becomes visible. Just seeing the single eye is not enough; it is more difficult for the devotee to go into that light. But by practice of the higher methods, the consciousness is led inside the spiritual eye, into another world of faster dimensions."

If I have lost you, just trust me for now. Dharana is a complete process, and with patience and faith, you too will experience this unity. I have often told my students to look for the light like you are looking out a portal in a spaceship into your own spirituality. Eventually it does lead you to a vastness like the universe.

As you focus, you smile with the joy of Jesus' presence and you pray. This is your time to talk and ask what is needed as well as give gratitude and thanksgiving for the past, present, and future. In pure dharana, it is impossible to truly pay attention and think of something else.

God wants you to talk to him like you would a friend. He wants to hear your requests, your worries, as well as, your praise and gratitude. Risk being honest, and expect his insight in return. You can always be "present" with God, no matter what is whirling around you.

After you have completed your prayer of needs and of thanksgiving, you could repeat over and over a mantra, or a short "prayer of the heart." A mantra consists of invoking the name of Christ to the deepest core of one's being. To invoke the name of Christ "in one's heart" is to call upon Him with the deepest intensity of faith.

If you want to gather all your desire into one simple word that the mind can easily retain, choose a short word rather than a long one. Fasten this word in your heart so that it never leaves you.

The continuous repetition helps unhook our minds of thoughts and images, that normally occupy our "monkey minds." Continually repeat your word (mantra) until you realize you are no longer speaking it and are in a truly mindless state. If your mind starts to wonder, renew the mantra again.

Recommended prayers:

"With love, my Lord, I pray." This can be shorten to "With love," "Lord," or "Love."

"Be still and know that I am God." Or just repeat over and over "Be still" and see Jesus' face.

"I love you with all my heart and soul, Lord." You can shorten to "All my heart and soul," "Love you," or "I Love you, Lord."

"Love and Peace, Lord." This can be translated to inhaling the word "Love" and exhaling "Peace."

The way to God is through Jesus. Jesus is shining brightly for us in dharana and dhyana. The light of Jesus shines in our mind like a beacon and eventually it shines even brighter in the presence of God.

+ Scripture References on Prayer

"Call to me and I will answer and reveal to you wondrous secrets that you haven't known" (Jeremiah 33:3).

"This is my prayer: that your love might become even more and more rich with knowledge and all kinds of insight. I pray this so that you will be able to decide what really matters and so you will be sincere and blameless on the day of Christ" (Philippians 1:9–11).

"But when you pray, go into your room, shut the door, and pray to your Father who is present in that secret place. Your Father who sees what you do in secret will reward you" (Matthew 6:6).

"Therefore I say to you, whatever you pray and ask for, believe that you will receive it, and it will be so for you. And whenever you stand up to pray, if you have something against anyone, forgive so that your Father in heaven may forgive your wrongdoings" (Mark 11: 24–25).

"Rejoice always. Pray continually. Give thanks in every situation because this is God's will for you in Christ Jesus" (I Thessalonians 5:16).

"So live in Christ Jesus the Lord in the same way as you received him. Be rooted and built up in him, be established in faith, and overflow with thanksgiving just as you were taught" (Colossians 2:6–7).

"Pursue the Lord and his strength; see his face always!" (I Chronicles 16:11).

"Answer me when I cry out, my righteous God! Set me free from my troubles! Have mercy on me! Listen to my prayer!" (Psalm 4:1).

"The Lord is far from the wicked, but he listens to the prayers of the righteous" (Proverbs 15:29).

Exercises:
- Keep a journal for two weeks of your dharana or prayer practice starting with three minutes and increase in one to two minute increments. Write down anything that comes up during the process. Remember, every day will be different, so be patient with yourself.
- Start a Prayer List.
- List five different activities that you could do off the mat to practice concentration.

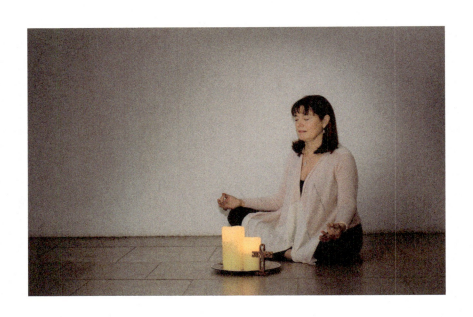

CHAPTER 8

The Seventh Limb of Yoga: Meditation or Dhyana

- ***Be Still and Listen***

We continue on this eight-faceted journey for the ultimate union with oneness with God. In the seventh of the Eight Limbs of Yoga is dhyana or mediation. The root of the practice is to cease all thinking and simply "be" with Christ. One way to think about meditation is that it is the practice of simply being light and love in the presence of Jesus.

Imagine being able to sit right in front of Jesus, looking him straight in the eyes to talk about things you are praying and grateful for, and then simply closing your eyes and being with him? This is true meditation.

We tend to be caught up in *doing* rather than *being*, in *action* rather than *awareness*. Psalm 46:10 reminds us, - "Be still, and know that I am God" (ESV). In these few words lies the key to the science of yoga. Silence is the language of the Spirit.

There are helpful tips for achieving dhyana. First of all, remember that meditation is difficult, and it is nearly impossible for a beginner to achieve complete meditation all at once. Meditation must be taken in, striven for, and then worked toward ardously.

Modern scientific research has proven that one of the most effective things anyone can do to promote mental and physical health is to sit quietly for 10 to 20 minutes a day. This is more effective than a change in diet, vitamins, food supplements, or medicines. It is not necessary to possess any special skill or training. All that is required is that one achieves a relaxed state of mind, unburdened by the thoughts of the day. For Christians, it is pausing in our hectic lives for time alone with God.

Meditation frees us from the personalities we wear. It is just God and us. There are no rules. This freedom can stay with us the rest of the day… in every action and every word. My experience during meditation is like peeling back layers and layers of roles I play… like an onion. During meditation I am not a mother, wife, friend, daughter, aunt, sister, or employee. What I feel is light, peace, love, and silence.

The ego does not like things to be simple. The ego will rebel in the beginning. Remember, meditation is actually our natural state. With time, meditation should feel comfortable and natural for you.

As I have previously stated, my thought has always been that praying is talking to God and meditation is listening to God. But it takes time, discipline, and devotion to truly create a meditation practice. Why? Because we all have such busy "monkey minds" that are constantly working, It takes time to quiet and calm down enough to truly let go of thoughts, words, and ideas. Remember, too, that we are "beings" not "doings." Start out with a simple five-minute meditation practice and gradually in increase overtime to 20-30 minutes each day. Meditation can change your life. Fact: Without inner peace, outer peace is impossible.

For Christians, Christ is the way to God. Pope John Paul II stated in his book, *Crossing the Threshold of Hope,* that, "Christ is absolutely original and absolutely unique. If He were a wise man like Socrates, if He were a "prophet" like Mohammed, if He were "enlightened" like Buddha, without any doubt He would not be what He is. He is the one mediator between God and humanity."

- *Be with Jesus*

At this point, we have withdrawn from our senses and allowed the Holy Spirit to enter our being. Next we have prayed to Jesus in a form of request and thanksgiving followed by a mantra, a short prayer of the heart.

Now, it is time to let go of our prayers to Jesus and simply "be." Visualize Jesus sitting in front of you and bask in His presence. Feel the tranquility and a heightened level of awareness without focus. In this state of tranquility, our minds should produce few or no thoughts at all. One must learn to meditate—how to switch off the attention from distractions of the senses, and learn how to keep the focus fixed on the spiritual eye where Christ can be received in all his glory—and then just be with Him.

+ **Scripture Reference for Meditation and Listening for the Lord**

"Jesus answered, "I am the way, the truth, and the life. No one comes to the Father except through me. If you have really known me, you will also know the Father. From now on you know him and have seen him" (John 14:6).

"Hope in the Lord! Be strong! Let your heart take courage! Hope in the Lord!" (Psalm 27:14).

"Don't suppress the Spirit. Don't brush off Spirit-inspired messages, but examine everything carefully and hang on to what is good" (I Thessalonians 5:17–21).

"During that time, Jesus went out to the mountain to pray, and he prayed to God all night long" (Luke 6:12).

"Jesus was telling them a parable about their need to pray continuously and not to be discouraged" (Luke 18:1).

"In the same way, the Spirit comes to help our weakness. We don't know what we should pray, but the Spirit himself pleads our case with unexpressed groans" (Romans 8:26).

"May the Lord cause you to increase and enrich your love for each other and for everyone in the same way as we also love you" (I Thessalonians 3:12).

"Keep on praying and guard your prayers with thanksgiving" (Colossians 4:14).

Exercises:
- What are the benefits of meditation? Look at other sources besides this book.
- Meditate a minimum of ten minutes a day for a week by just being still with your eyes closed. See if you can work up to twenty minutes.

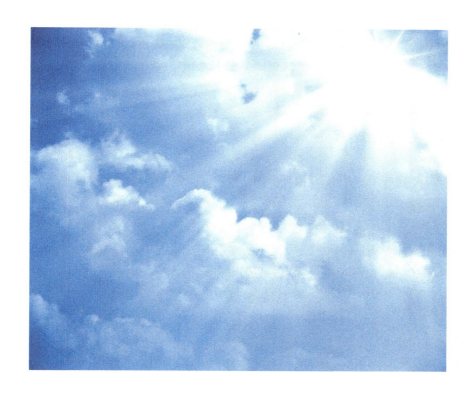

CHAPTER 9

The Eight Limb of Yoga: Oneness with God (Samadhi)

Samadhi is the highest step on the Eightfold Path of Yoga. It follows dhyana, or the meditation and stillness with Jesus. Samadhi is an intense state of meditation, commonly referred to as the union with the Divine or oneness with God. You have experienced Jesus by going to your own center of being, and you are now ready to pass through it into the center of God.

The Eighth Limb of Yoga is connected to the crown chakra (more on the chakras in Chapter 10), where a shining, bright light stems from the top of your head and reaches up to the heavens and your Higher Source. Samadhi urges you to escape from worldly troubles and enter into your original innocent self of pure joy. There you will bask in the brightness of the Lord.

Jesus described this journey with such beautiful conciseness when he explained that freedom means "being in the world but not of it." Joy with detachment is the spiritual aim of life and a part of the yoga journey. On the yoga path, you will experience moments of both, and there will be stretches when neither is possible. Your ego will shout its demands, and the "I, me and mine" will have to be tended to. This is natural. Be patient... but persevere.

- ***Be One with God***

Through meditation and being with Jesus, you are now ready to find oneness with God.

Shift your attention to the crown of your head. Visualize a bright light shining from your skull into the heavens. Reflect on the brightness and the joy of being one with God. There is no separation. Allow yourself to feel the ultimate bliss in the oneness with the Father, Son, and Holy Ghost.

This state can be accomplished by anyone who follows the Eight Limbs of Yoga with patience, consistency, faith, and the love of God. You will also learn to find God in all things in order to love and serve God in all things. God is always "at home" in us; it is we who are usually absent. A single moment of absorption in God is more valuable than a longer period of prayer during which we are constantly in and out of inner silence.

One cannot expect quick results on this path. There is no "instant yoga." Samadhi sometimes requires a continuous and uninterrupted number of years to achieve. Commit and you will be rewarded. It is a path of joy and bliss.

Step-by-Step Summary to Your Daily Meditation Practice

1. Set aside ten to thirty minutes a day, preferably in the morning, to be still.

Find a quiet place in your home for your daily meditation. Turn your cell phone off, shut the door, make sure the pets are in another room, etc. Then get into as comfortable sitting position as possible, whether on a chair or on the floor, with your spine straight. Keeping your spine straight is an essential element of meditation to ensure there is no resistance in your body's flow of energy.

2.   Close your eyes and allow the Holy Spirit to fill you.

Sit still and upright, relaxed but alert, with your eyes lightly closed. Begin withdrawing from all your senses and go deeper and deeper within. Allow the Holy Spirit to fill you.

3.   Take your attention to your "third" eye.

Draw your attention internally to the space between your two eyebrows. Focusing internally on this "third eye" will be like looking through a *porthole* into your spirituality. When your mind is still, you will be able to discover this space with awe. Your vision through the porthole might be like looking into the darkness of the universe where the spaciousness of infinity is miraculous. As thoughts come up, you will just recognize them as clouds passing by in the sky. Stay focused and concentrate on that space. This is the door to the kingdom of God.

4.   Look for the Light

When the eyes are focused and still, and the breath and mind are calm, a light begins to form in the forehead. The vibrating light will lead you to Christ.

5.   Pray and Talk to God

Pray for everyone that comes into your thoughts. Praise God for all the blessings in your life and ask God for help with any needs you have or any trials you may be going through.

Internally begin to say a single word or phrase selected from the context of your Christian faith. This word or phrase can be your mantra. Listen to it as you gently but continuously speak those words with faith and love. If thoughts or images come and your attention strays, as soon as you become aware of this, return to saying your word or phrase.

6.   Concentration will lead to meditation where you will be in a place of just being with God.

Let all internal focus and prayer go. You have reached dhyana where true meditation will take place. Be still and smile. You are in the presence of our Lord, Jesus Christ.

Spiritual truth and wisdom are found in the "wilderness" of inner silence. You will find the answers to all the questions in your heart. Listen and be still.

"If we're not trying to hold on to the past, and not jockeying into a position for the future, then we finally belong in the world as it exists in the present moment, the eternal "Now" (Bo Lozoff).

7. Feel the bliss.

Now turn your attention to the crown of your head, the seventh chakra, and see a bright light shining from your skull to the heavens. You are no longer separate from God but one. This is samadhi, the highest limb of yoga. With time your meditation practice will lead to a feeling of oneness with God. You go so deep that you feel you *are* one with God. *The Kingdom of God is the midst of you"* Luke 17:21 (ESV).

You will find a state of bliss, a joy that never grows stale. Bliss is a much deeper state than peace. It is a sin (a word I don't use lightly) to think that there is no chance of being happy, to abandon all hope of attaining peace. Bliss is the irrevocable divine birthright of every soul.

Our true nature is joy. You should settle for nothing less, and you can find it again and again through meditation. Let your heart dwell on the Lord, and let nothing else distract you.

8. Leave in peace

When you are ready to come out of your meditation slowly give thanks for your practice... for the joy, peace, and love that are the benefits of meditation. End with *The Prayer of Jabez:*

> *Oh, that You would bless me indeed,*
> *and enlarge my territory,*
> *that Your hand would be with me,*
> *and that You would keep me from evil,*
> *that I may not cause pain.*

By praying the *Prayer of Jabez*, you ask every day to be blessed! You will see your "territory" expand in so many ways. Ask God then to lead you, especially in times when you know you are out of your comfort zone. This is the only way you will grow spiritually. During the process, ask God to keep you from evil and that you should cause no pain.

As Bruce Wilkinson wrote in the book, *The Prayer of Jabez,* this prayer will change your life. Mine did. You will be sending out joy and peace to your friends and fellow yogis. Doors will open up like never before. To pray for larger borders is to ask for a miracle—it's that simple. A miracle is something that happens which we may not expect or understand, but nevertheless, reminds us of God's active presence in our world..

Be patient and consistent in dedicating 10-30 minutes a day to a meditation practice. Some days you will find that your mind will quiet down in seconds where as other days it might take 30 minutes. Learn to be with God—that is the be-all and end-all of life. Effort is necessary. He *is* within you. Every grain of food you eat, every breath you take, is God. Think of Him all the time—before you act, while you are engaged in activity, and after activity. We often pray to God before a certain action for guidance but then forget to thank him afterwards. As we end this section—thank you, God, with all my heart and soul.

+ Scriptures for Bliss and Oneness with God (Samadhi)

"But your loyal love, Lord, extends to the skies; your faithfulness reaches the clouds" (Psalm 36:5).

"Therefore, humble yourselves under God's power so that he many raise you up in the last day. Throw all your anxiety onto him, because he cares about you" (I Peter 5:6–7).

"All the people were beside themselves with wonder. Filled with awe, they glorified God, saying 'We've seen unimaginable things today" (Luke 15:26).

"You teach me the way of life. In your presence is total celebration. Beautiful things are always in your right hand" (Psalm 16:11).

"He took me in a Spirit-inspired trance to a great, high mountain, and he showed me the holy city, Jerusalem, coming down out of heaven from God" (Revelation 21:10).

"Dear friends, now we are God's children, and it hasn't yet appeared what we will be. We know that when He appears we will be like Him because we'll see Him as He is. And everyone who has this hope in Him purifies himself even as He is pure" (I John 3: 2–3).

"The grace of God has appeared, bringing salvation to all people. It educates us so that we can live sensible, ethical, and godly lives right now by rejecting ungodly lives and the desires of the world. At the same time we wait for the blessed hope and the glorious appearance of our Great God and savior Jesus Christ" (Titus 1:11–13).

Exercises:
- What would/does Samadhi look like to you?
- What do you think heaven will be like?
- In your own words, what is the true purpose of yoga?
- Give two additional scriptures that you believe resonate with the limb of blissfulness with God.

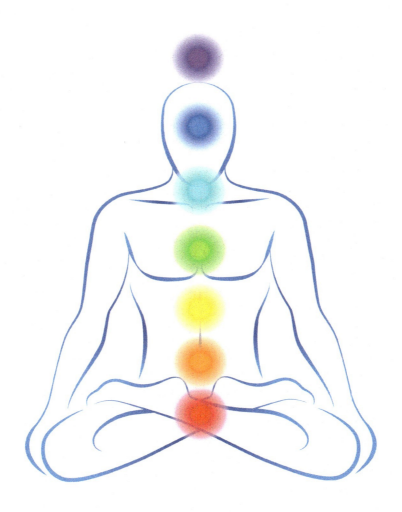

CHAPTER 10

Seven Ways to Create Balance and Healing via the Chakras

All of us may, at one time or another, feel unbalanced in areas of our lives. These areas might eventually create a disconnect to the world around us, feeling a lack of creativity and sexuality, a loss of personal power, not feeling love or compassion, not communicating effectively, getting headaches regularly, or not feeling oneness with a higher source.

Chakras are the human energy centers of the body. Many people around the world are turning to chakra healing as an alternative to mainstream medicine. Chakras are energy centers that run from the base of the spine out the top, or crown, of the head. The word chakra is a Sanskrit word, meaning wheel or disc. There are seven major chakras, each a circular wheel of light spinning in a person's energetic system. Blocked energy in any of the seven chakras can often lead to illness, so it is important to understand what each chakra represents and what can be done to keep this energy flowing freely.

Each chakra is associated with specific body parts, a color, a sense, gemstones, aromatherapy, element, and function. By learning to tune into the energy of one's chakra, a person can begin to embrace the fullness of their being.

Most importantly, opening up chakras will facilitate the Ajna Chakra or "third eye" (enabling the individual to see Jesus more clearly) and the Crown Chakra to connect and bring oneness with God.

Here's a quick summary of the Seven Chakras:

1. **Root or Muladhara Chakra** – Represents our foundation and feeling of being grounded. It governs our most basic survival needs.

   Location: Base of spine in pelvic area, including legs and feet.

   Emotional issues: Survival issues, such as finances, independence, money, and food.

   Blockage creates anxiety, worry, apathy, and lack of trust. Basic needs like food, shelter, and water are necessary in order for this chakra to feel balanced.

   Open creates stability, confidence, serenity, and a sense of belonging.

   Color: Red

   Element: Earth

   Sense: Smell

   Scent: Patchouli

   Stones: Ruby, Bloodstone, Garnet, Red Jasper

   Mantra: Lam

2. **Sacral or Svadhisthana Chakra** – Our seat of creativity, joy, enthusiasm, sexuality, and sensuality.

   Location: Lower abdomen near the reproductive organ.

   Emotional issues: Sense of abundance, well-being, pleasure, and sexuality.

   Blockage causes one to be stiff and unemotional, causing the person to be closed off from others.

   Open frees the emotional and physical flow, fuels the creative force to paint, write, etc. resulting in one being happily connected to life.

   Color: Orange

   Element: Water

   Sense: Taste

Scent: Sandalwood or Ylang Ylang
Stones: Golden Topaz, Citrine, Gold Calcite
Mantra: Vam

3. **Naval or Manipura Chakra** – The seat of our personal sense of power, our ability to be confident and in-control of our lives.
Location: Upper abdomen in the stomach area/Solar plexus
Emotional issues: Self-worth, self-confidence, and self-esteem.
Blockage causes individuals to be either too aggressive or too passive and blame others for what is bogging them down.
Open enables the implementation of intentions with assertiveness and to feel worthy of all that life has to offer.
Color: Yellow
Element: Fire
Sense: Sight
Scent: Cinnamon or Peppermint
Stones: Topaz, Yellow Citrine, Amber, Tiger's Eye
Mantra: Ram

4. **Heart or Anahata Chakra** – Our seat of love and compassion. Clarifies that the relationship between the physical heart and the emotional heart is more than metaphorical. The more we love, the healthier we are.
Location: Center of chest just above heart, and including arms and hands.
Emotional issues: Love, joy, inner peace.
Blockage gives the feeling of alienation.
Open connects to others from an understanding, considerate, and peaceful place.
Color: Green
Element: Air
Sense: Touch
Scent: Rose

Stones: Emerald, Green Jade, Rose Quartz, Green or Pink
  Tourmaline
Mantra: Yum

5. **Throat or Vishuddha Chakra** – Our seat of communication and truth.
Location: Throat.
Emotional issues: Communication, self-expression of feelings, the truth.
Blockage gives a feeling of not being heard. Often a connected to thyroid problems or chronic neck pain.
Open allows easy communication and articulation.
Color: Light blue
Element: Ether/Space
Sense: Hearing
Scent: Eucalyptus
Stones: Turquoise, Blue Agate, Aquamarine, Blue Topaz
Mantra: Hum

6. **Third Eye or Ajna Chakra** – Our seat of intuition and perception. It is also our ability to focus on and see the big picture.
Location: Forehead between the eyes.
Emotional issues: Intuition, imagination, wisdom, ability to think and make decisions.
Blockage stops the individual from being open to seeing Jesus.
Open helps focus on the front of the brain which serves as a portal to spirituality. Enables a clear sense of *dharma* or life's purpose.
Color: Indigo blue
Element: ---
Sense: Inner Sounds
Scent: Lavender
Stones: Sapphire, Tanzanite, Lapis Lazuli, Clear Quartz
Mantra: Sham or OM

7. **Crown or Sahaswara Chakra** – The highest Chakra represents our ability to be fully connected spiritually.
   Location: The very top of the head.
   Emotional issues: Inner and outer beauty, our connection to spirituality; pure bliss.
   Blockage prevents one from seeing the bright light shining up to the heavens.
   Open allows oneness with God.
   Color: Violet or bright white
   Element: ---
   Sense: Inner Light
   Scent: Frankincense
   Stones: Amethyst, Diamond, Purple Fluorite
   Mantra: OM

When roots are receiving nourishment from the earth in the first chakra…

> … the creative juices flow in the second
> … the intentions are empowered in the third
> … the heart is open and exchanges love with others in the fourth
> … leading to expressing one's highest self in the fifth
> … bringing one in touch with the inner voice in the sixth
> … then the energy moves into the crown chakra, reminding the person of their essential nature as infinite and unbounded.

"The thousand-petal lotus flower unfolds"; the person understands the meaning of a spiritual being temporarily localized to a body and mind. The person is connected to God as one.

From the time of birth, we have been called to explore the world outside of us. Meditation is the exploration of our inner world. Yoga encourages us to be as familiar with that inner world of thoughts, feelings, memories, desires, and imagination as we live within the outer world of time, space, and causality.

Everything we need to know is inside of us. Each of us has all of the answers to all of the questions that we ask. What is needed is to slow down, take some time out, listen and trust in our own wisdom.

Exercise:

Who am I? Make a list under each category of words that described you at that time in your life. Words like: girl/boy, daughter/son, elementary/middle school, outgoing/shy, etc.

- Root Chakra – Womb to twelve months
- Sacral Chakra – Six months to two years
- Manipura Chakra – Eighteen months to four years
- Heart Chakra – Four to seven years old
- Throat Chakra – Seven to twelve years old
- Ajna Chakra –Adolescent
- Crown – Rest of your adult life

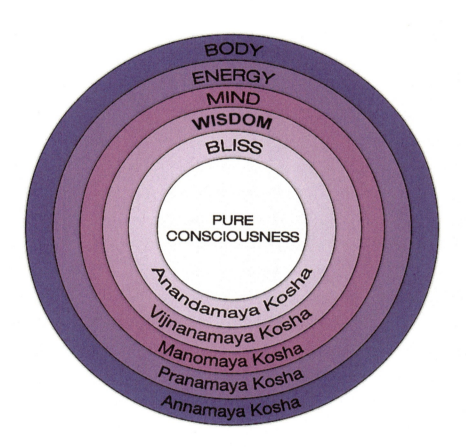

CHAPTER 11

The Five Koshas – Layers of Your Being

The Five Kosha model, along with the Chakras, gives a structure to make sure we are living a balanced life. In layman's term, a balanced life is being physically, emotionally, mentally, socially, and spiritually fulfilled. The Koshas follow a similar format and helps us to understand ourselves and others.

The koshas also provide a map to follow into our true self. It helps us recognize that we are multilayered, multidimensional beings. The layers are interdependent in varying degrees. We are a brilliant kaleidoscope of body, mind, thoughts, emotions, wisdom, and bliss. Our yoga practices help nourish, cleanse, and balance each kosha, and direct all of our layers toward harmony.

The Five Koshas are:

Annamaya Kosha	**Physical layer**	**Body**
Pranamaya Kosha	**Energy layer**	**Breath/Life Force**
Manomaya Kosha	**Mental layer**	**Mind/Emotions**
Vijnanamaya Kosha	**Intellect layer**	**Wisdom**
Anandamaya Kosha	**Bliss layer**	**Bliss**

Annamaya Kosha represents our physical body, including the skin, muscles, fat, bones, and connective tissues. It is also the physical realm all around us—it's what we see, taste, feel, smell, and hear. All that we experience physically is annamaya kosha, which thrives on healthy food and loves asana and pranayama.

Pranamaya Kosha represents the vital body. In essence, it is the circulatory system for *prana,* or "life-force energy." Prana is carried by the breath. It is abundant in healthy natural environments and organic produce, and is depleted in polluted environments and junk food. It is easy to imagine the full range of *pranic* situations—good and bad. Prana is the organizing field that holds the material body together and governs biological processes from breathing to digestion to circulation.

Manomaya Kosha is the part of us that takes in information from the outside via the five senses. It is our capacity to learn. This layer takes us into the deep recesses of the mind, emotions, and nervous system. All the functions of the brain are within this kosha. It's this layer where we move from physical feeling to emotional feeling.

Vijnanamaya Kosha is our power of judgment and intellect as well as the layer that develops wisdom and insight. We gain insights through self-reflection and understanding of subtler realms. This is the realm that separates us from other animals, since it allows us to direct our lives and make moral choices. We develop this part of ourselves through embodying the yamas and ni-yamas. The study of knowledge in Jnana Yoga also helps with this development. (The word jnana means wisdom and is the root of "vijnanamaya"). Vijnanamaya kosha is nourished by spiritual understandings and ideas.

"What of the wisdom from above? First, it is pure, and then peaceful, gentle, obedient, filled with mercy and good actions, fair, and genuine" (James 3:17).

Anandamaya Kosha drops from conscious awareness into a pure and radiant bliss within the body. Bliss is our true nature. The very core of our being is joy. We can experience love as God loves—with unspeakable intensity. We nourish this layer by selfless service, which opens our heart to others. Bhakti yoga, or devotion to God, and Samadhi, intense meditation, opens our heart to love, joy, and bliss. And, Anandamaya kosha thrives on bliss! Undernourishment feels like lack of purpose or spiritual fulfillment. Experiencing joy, pure joy, for no reason is the fulfillment of anandamaya kosha.

Throughout the day, notice the shifting between the koshas layers.

A poetic expression from the *Taittiriya Upanishad*: (6th century) beautifully explains the Koshas.

> *"Human beings consist of a material body built from the food they eat. Those who care for this body are nourished by the universe itself."*
>
> *"Inside this is another body made of life energy. It fills the physical body and takes its shape. Those who treat this vital force as divine experience obtains longevity because this energy is the source of physical life."*
>
> *"Within the vital force is yet another body, this one made of thought energy. It fills the two denser bodies and has the same shape. Those who understand and control the mental body are no longer afflicted by fear."*
>
> *"Deeper still lays another body comprised of intellect. It permeates the three denser bodies and assumes the same form. Those who establish their awareness here free themselves from unhealthy thought and action and develops the self-control necessary to achieve their goals."*
>
> *"Hidden inside it is yet a subtler body, composed of pure joy. It pervades the other bodies and shares the same shape. It is experienced as happiness, delight, and bliss."*

Pain Can Affect Your Psyche

One beautiful fall afternoon as I was trail riding through the woods, my horse got spooked by a buck that was charging over a fence and jumping into a nearby pond. Maverick reared up perpendicular to the earth. I had no choice but to let go of the reins seven feet in the air and land flat on my back. He then fell on his back missing me by inches. Fortunately, only the breath was knocked out of me. I got up and walked both of us back to the barn, thanking God that I could.

Unfortunately, two months later I woke up to a sciatic nerve problem from my lower back and down my left leg. Some days I considered the pain to be a ten on a scale of one to ten. Thus began my journey of recovery that included yoga, chiropractic sessions, acupuncture, physical therapy, and massage.

Pain can be debilitating in may ways. The yoga concept of koshas did not really resonate with me while going through yoga teacher training 14 years ago. As I began meditating on this topic of physical pain during this time period and what it does to the rest of the psyche, I began to understand this powerful concept of koshas. Yoga improves the physical body, but it is also comprised of techniques that act on the mind and emotions, and provides a complete philosophy of living. It can also be used as a method of self-study.

Yoga practioners believe that there are five layers or sheaths of energy that confine the spirit or essential self. These five layers, called koshas, are the physical body, the mind, the breath/energy, the intellect and the bliss/spiritual. My experience taught me when there is physical pain, the other layers are also out of whack. It was hard for me to focus mentally when I was constantly aware of my physical pain.

I continued my bodywork appointments to help fix my sciatic problem. I gradually got 95 percent back to my normal self before I then headed to Costa Rica to lead a yoga, adventure, and service retreat. Prior to my group arriving, I joined a separate meditation group for a few days.

It is there that I meditated on these five levels of the self. I wanted to find gratitude by focusing separately on each kosha. I began by thanking God for my physical capabilities and committed again to treating my body as a temple through healthy food, exercise, and rest. Gratitude along with understanding came when meditating on the pranayama (or breath/life energy) kosha. I learned when I did have pain to acknowledge it without being consumed by it. The breath sheath is just as important as the physical body and gives the emotional energy needed. Mentally, I was grateful for my mind and vowed to keep it healthy through positive thinking and new experiences. The intellect or wisdom sheath seemed to be assembling the connection of the five sheaths for me. It was a "light bulb" moment for me. When focus began on the "bliss" sheath, I expected it to be a separate experience such as what deep meditation can bring, but it was not a separate feeling. Rather, it seemed like a natural connection of all five layers of my being that were present and completely working together. Our soul or self consists of all these layers, and we should be consciously aware that all should be balanced and healthy. The bottom line: We are NOT our pain, our cancer, our disability… Physical ailments do not define who we are. Yoga helps develop the ability to maintain inner peace at all times. According to the ultimate yogi book, *The Yoga Sutras*, it is our God-given right to find bliss. Now who wouldn't want that?

Exercise:

How do the koshas resonate with you regarding the practice of Yoga through Christ? How can you use them in your own life? Identify ways to begin incorporating the five koshas into your practice.

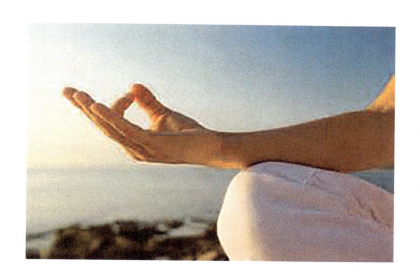

CHAPTER 12

Mudras and Aromatherapy

Mudras are hand postures, commonly referred to as hand yoga, that are directly related to the energy flow in the human body. In Sanskrit, the word *mudra* means "closure" or "seal" meaning that mudras are used in a way to lock and guide energy through the body. Mudras are a silent language or self-expression used most commonly during meditation and pranayama. This ancient practice of yoga is a way to link the mind to the energy of the body.

Using mudras during yoga is encouraged because they provide physical, mental, and spiritual benefits. The basic idea of using mudras is that each finger is correlated to one of the five vital body elements: earth, wind, fire, water, and ether. Deficiencies or an excess of any element can cause a disorder and imbalance in the mind and body, therefore the curling, crossing, stretching, and touching of the five fingers are a way to balance these elements. The five fingers are related to the five elements as follows:

- Thumb: Fire
- Index Finger: Air
- Middle Finger: Ether
- Ring Finger: Earth
- Pinky: Water

By gently pressing into the fingers, but not enough to whiten the fingertips, the elements are able to be balanced and different emotions/concepts are provoked. Mudras should be held for at least several minutes. Holding the mudras with both hands makes the effects more powerful and keeps balance in the body.

Padma Mudra: Love and Compassion

Instructions: Mimics a blossoming flower – connect the thumbs and pinkies to one another with the outer edges of the hands sealed together, splay the rest of the fingers outward. Hold the opening of the hands near the heart and below the chin.

Benefits: Opens the heart center, cultivating an experience of love and compassion, an open-hearted acceptance of ourselves, others, and life.

Vajrapadama Mudra: Unshakable Confidence

Instructions: Interlace the fingers with the palms spread apart facing the heart and the thumbs up.

Benefits: Instills a sense of unshakable trust and confidence that unfolds from within, a knowing that life supports us unconditionally.

Garuda Mudra: Spiritual Transformation

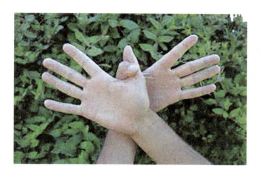

Instructions: Cross the thumbs in front of the heart with the palms of the hands facing toward the heart center and fingers spread open like wings.

Benefits: Evokes the experience of spiritual awakening, a feeling of lightness and joy that are reflections of our true nature.

Adhi Mudra: Grounding and Security

Instructions - Place the thumbs into the palms of the hands and fold the other fingers around them forming a fist. Rest the hands, palms down onto the thighs.

Benefits: Cultivates a deep sense of grounding as if rooted to the earth and a sense of security, knowing that all that is needed is already present in this moment.

Jnana Mudra: Wisdom

Instructions - Touch the tip of the thumb to the tip of the index finger forming a circle. The other three fingers are extended straight out.

Benefits: Increases concentration and memory, ability to cure insomnia and symbols oneness with God.

The steps to using mudras are quite simple. Sit with a straight back in comfortable seated position and place the hands in the chosen position. Close your eyes. Often people accompany the mudra with a mantra such as "Be Still." After practicing the mudra for at least a few minutes, release the hands and slowly open the eyes.

Mudras provide many benefits to the body, especially allowing the life force to flow freely to various body parts. It has been said the entire universe lies within our ten fingers.

Aromatherapy

During the thirty years I was in the corporate world, I would often keep a bottle of lavender on my desk. Periodically, I would take a whiff to de-stress and center myself. It worked... plus it reminded me of France, which would always bring a smile to my face.

Certain essential oils can trigger physical or emotional effects on their own. For instance, lavender is a widely known calming agent, whereas peppermint is a mood lifter.

Inhaling essential oils transmits messages to a part of the brain responsible for controlling emotions and influencing the nervous system. These messages are believed to affect factors such as heart rate, stress levels, blood pressure, insomnia, depression, breathing, and immune function.

Here is a list of some popular oils and their benefits:

- **Lavender** – The Healer. A versatile, relaxing, skin-loving property with beautiful floral fragrance makes it one of the most popular essential oil. Often called "The First Aid Kit in a Bottle." It is used for restlessness, insomnia, nervousness, depression, and even can be used on common cuts, bruises, and skin irritations. According to Rev. Janet McBride (*Scriptural Essence*), lavender was used in worship by Moses and the priests in the Old Testament.
- **Frankincense** – Spiritual Awakener. Known to be the holy anointing oil in the Middle East, it has been used in religious ceremonies for thousands of years. It was one of the gifts to Jesus from the Wise Men. Useful for visualizing, improving one's spiritual connection, and centering, it has comforting properties that help focus the mind and overcome stress and despair.
- **Peppermint** – Digestion Soother. One of the oldest and most highly regarded herbs for soothing digestion and nausea. A type of mint was found in Egyptian tombs dating to 1000 BC. Peppermint clears the mind and refreshes the spirit.

- **Rose** – Mood Lifter. Helpful in times of stress, it is the oil of choice for times of grief, depression, and anxiety. Rose essential oil has been used throughout history in the ancient art of aromatherapy as a healing tonic and mood-elevating supplement.
- **Thieves** – Immune Protector. Legend tells of four infamous thieves in France who protected themselves from the Black Plague with a combination of cloves, rosemary, and other scents while they robbed victims of the killer disease. When captured, they were offered a lighter sentence in exchange for their secret recipe. It is highly effective in supporting the immune system and good health.

Many of the above suggestions along with many other oils were used in ancient practices that have diminished with time. Today, there has been a resurging interest in these natural oils for healing and health. In addition, stress has been strongly connected to disease, and certain essential oils, like rose and lavender, can be beneficial in being proactive in prevention of illness.

Thomas Edison penned it correctly when he wrote, *"The doctor of the future will give no medicine, but will interest his patients in the care of the human frame, in diet, and in the cause and prevention of disease.*

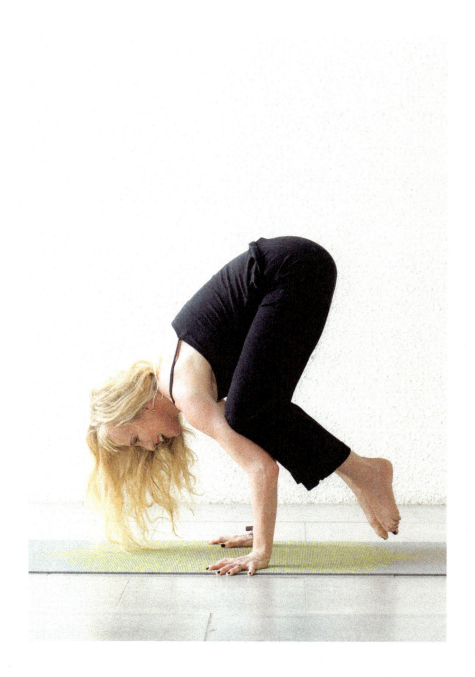

CHAPTER 13

A Class Template

Yoga through Christ
(Via the Eight Limbs of Yoga)

- First and Second Limbs – select a *Yama* and/or *Ni-Yama/*
  Social and Personal Observances – ***Set an Intention with***
  Scripture and Prayer

  Example of Intention: ***Truth***
  "Little children, let's not love with words or speech but with
  action and truth" (1 John 3:18).

- Third Limb – *Asana/*Physical Practice – ***Prayerful Movement***
- Fourth Limb – *Pranayama/*Breath Control – ***Breathe for***
  Peace and Love

  "Let every living thing praise the Lord!" (Psalm 150:6).

- Fifth Limb – *Pratyahara/*Withdrawal from the Senses – ***Go***
  Inward
- Sixth Limb – *Dhyana/*Concentration – ***Pray***
- Seventh Limb – *Dhyana/*Meditation – ***BE with Jesus***

"Be still, and know that I am God" (Psalm 46:10, ESV).

Silence can be uncomfortable, but being uncomfortable is necessary for both our spiritual and physical lives. Therefore, in this moment, we sit in silence. We sit in solidarity. Offering ourselves fully to God by listening for the still, small voice that transforms and heals us each and every day.

- Eighth Limb – *Samadhi*/Bliss – **Be ONE with God**
- Savasana – Let go, let God. Leave everything on the mat that no longer serves you. Celebrate this time of rebirth and renewal.
- Jabez's Prayer: *May you be blessed, may your territories be expanded, may you be directed, may you be kept from evil, and may you cause no pain.*
- OM to go Home.

For Teachers
The Class Template – (75-minute Practice)
Ambiance (Optional ideas)

- Students enter in silence
- Optional class program can be given regarding the Eight Limbs of Yoga
- Christian instrumental music played throughout class
- Teacher could wear all white
- Room is semi-dark and candles are lit
- Mats are set up in a circle around the room
- Gong or bowl can be used when it is time to move from one limb to another
- Have some type of essential oil, such as frankincense, to place between each student's eyebrows as they are laying on the mat
- 50 percent or more of any proceeds from the class goes to charity

Flow of Class

Use the sound of the gong or bowl to call class to begin. Students sit in easy pose with eyes closed and hands in jnana mudra. Leader leads them through centering, letting go of thoughts, and awareness of breath. Explain the Ujjayi or Victorious Breath to use throughout the class.

- Choose a Yama or Niyama based on scripture and read to the class
- Lead the "Yoga through Christ" asana flow. Use essential oils, such as frankincense, lavender, or peppermint.
- Demonstrate and lead Ego Eradicator Pranayama (rapid exhales with arms lifted in a V and thumbs pointed to the heavens) and Alternating Nostril Breathing (five to eight full rounds)
- Invite the students to find a meditative seated position that will work for them the next ten to twenty minutes (time will vary depending on longevity of the class). Instruct the students to close their eyes, withdraw from their senses, and fill their bodies by breathing in the Holy Spirit, going deeper and deeper with each breath.
- With the students' eyes closed explain the three final Limbs of Yoga and explain that a tap on the gong or bowl will indicate to move on to the next step. Determine the amount of time for each of the three limbs based on the meditation level the class.

    • Dharana or concentration on Jesus begins by drawing one's attention to the Third Eye and praying. Talk to God. After completing your prayers of request or thanksgiving, continuously repeat a brief prayer. Suggest a word or phrase for the individuals who do not have their own. For example: Love and peace, my Lord. Or inhale in "love" and exhale "peace." After approximately three minutes or more, use the gong or bowl to move to the 7th Limb of Yoga.
    • Dharma or Meditation – Be still and be with God. This timeframe can be three to ten minutes depend-

ing on the class. Remind students that if their mind wanders to bring the attention back to the breath.

- Samadhi or Oneness with God begins by turning our inward attention to the crown of the head and visualizing a bright light. This bright light will shine up to the heavens mixing with an even brighter light. There brilliance and a feeling of bliss will be found. Put a smile on your face and bask in the oneness with God. This can also be three to ten minutes.

- The final gong invites the students to lay down in savasana with their ankles crossed and their arms directly out to their sides, symbolizing Jesus on the cross. This pose is called corpse, and it encourages students to leave anything on the mat that no longer serves them in their walk of faith.
- After four to eight minutes in savasana, the students are invited to roll to one side and curl up in a ball. This is the fetal position representing rebirth and renewal.
- After approximately a minute or two, ask the students to return to a seated position with their eyes closed.
- End with a prayer or a song.

Peace...
be on my heart
around my thoughts
through my words
with my actions
each minute
every day
all day throughout the year.

Om shanti, shanti, shanti
Om peace, peace, peace.

- OM to go Home.

Summary

Yoga is a way to seek, be silent, wait, and obey by living a life that God desires for each of us. A famous Chinese Proverb reminds us of what can happen when we practice yoga with a spiritual heart and truly seek to a abide in Christ.

"What I hear, I forget.
What I see, I remember.
What I do, I know."

Max Lucado eloquently wrote in his book, *Grace for the Moment*, "We think of God as a deity to discuss, not a place to dwell. We think of God as a mysterious miracle worker, not a house to live in. We think of God as a creator to call on, not a home to reside in. But our Father wants to be much more. He wants us to be like Acts 17:28, the one in whom we live and move and have our being."

In the words of BKS Iyengar, "In the spiritual world as in the physical, one can climb a mountain from various directions. One way may be long, another short, one winding and difficult, another straightforward and easy, yet by all these paths it is possible to reach the summit."

May the practice of *Yoga through Christ* become a way to worship God. Striving to be Christ-like through yoga enables individuals to truly worship while finding joy, peace, and love in their hearts.

From all the teachings in the Bible, LOVE is what God fervently desires for our whole being. "I give you a new commandment: Love each other. Just as I have loved you, so you also must love each other. This is how everyone will know that you are my disciples, when you love each other" John 13:34. Through an intentional Christian yoga practice, we can work towards more fully achieving this command.

No yoga. No peace. Know yoga. Know peace.

We end with a closing word:

Yoga classes end with the word "Namaste", which means the light in me honors the light in you. Namaste is translated here with a Christian emphasis, "I honor the light in you as you honor the light in me, and together, we share the light of Christ to the world."

Together we say… Namaste!

RECOMMENDED READINGS

1. *Common English Bible* – a fresh translation to touch the heart and mind (Harrisburg, PA: Church Publishing Incorporated, 2013)
2. Bethany B. Connelly, *Finding Jesus on the Mat: Your Yoga Daily Devotional* (2012)
3. BKS Iyengar, *The Tree of Yoga,* (Boston, Massachusetts: Shambhala Publications, Inc., 1988)
4. Gary Kraftsow, *Yoga for Transformation,* (New York, New York: Penguin Compass, 2002)
5. Leonard Perlmutter, *Heart and Science of Yoga,* (Averill Park, New York: AMI Publishers, 2005)
6. Thomas Ryan, *Prayer of Heart and Body – Meditation and Yoga as Christian Spiritual Practice* (Mahwah, New Jersey: Paulist Press, 1995)
7. Sri Swami Satchidananda, *The Yoga Sutras of Patanjali* (Yogaville, Virginia: Integral Yoga Publications, 1978)
8. Mukunda Stiles, *Yoga Sutras of Patanjali* (Boston, MA: Weiser Books, 2002)
9. Bruce Wilkinson, *The Prayer of Jabez* (Sisters, Oregon: Multnomah Publishers, Inc., 2000)
10. Paramahansa Yogananda, *The Yoga of Jesus* (United States: Self-Realization Fellowship, 2007)

ACKNOWLEDGMENTS

Special thanks to my Bhakti yoga friends (lovers of God) for their support and input—Evelyn Byerly, Jan Dorsey, Diane Mitchell, Larry Morwick and Chris Yovanovich. (The latter is also the lovely model throughout the book). As always, I am grateful to my incredible husband, Dennis, for his support and encouragement, as well as, to my two beautiful daughters, Ashley and Laura, who also enjoy getting on the mat. Last, but never least, I thank our Heavenly Father for this amazing journey. Namaste!

GLOSSARY

AHIMSA – The practice of non-violence in thought, word, or deed.

AJNA CHAKRA – The sixth chakra, located between the eye brows and often referred at the "third eye". This is the seat of intuition and perception. It is also our ability to focus on and see the big picture.

ANAHATA CHAKRA – The heart chakra is the seat of love and compassion. A relationship between the physical heart and the emotional heart is more than metaphorical. The more you love, the healthier you are.

APARIGRAHA – The practice of non-attachment or non-greediness. This particular principle emphasizes being truly happy with what we have. It is not about searching for that happiness through possessions or another individual.

AROMATHERAPY – The practice of using natural oils to enhance psychological and physical well-being.

ASANAS – The yoga poses or postures that assist in creating strength, endurance, flexibility, and balance to eventually prepare the body for extended periods of meditation.

ASTEYA – The practice of non-stealing.

BHAGAVAD GITA – A core text of Indian philosophy.

BHAKTI YOGA – The path of devotion and intense love for God. It has been called "love for love's sake".

BRAMACHARYA – This is the practice of moderation (sometimes referred to as sexual purity). It requires self-restraint in order to use energy toward spiritual and devotional practices. The word translations to alk with God".

CHAKRAS – This term refers to wheels of energy throughout the body. There are seven main chakras, which align the spine, starting from the base of the spine through to the crown of the head. Each of the chakras contains our psychological, emotional, and spiritual states of being. It's essential that our chakras stay open, aligned, and fluid. If there is a blockage, energy cannot flow.

DHARANA – This is the practice of concentration and drawing the senses to a singular object or focus. The mind concentrates without wavering and avoids all other thoughts. As a Christian, the focus would be on Jesus.

DHARMA – This term refers to an individual's moral and religious duty, as well as their life's purpose. Dharma also represents the right way of living.

DHYANA – This is the state of profound meditation. The root of the practice is when we cease all thinking and simply "be". One way to think about meditation is that it is the practice of simply being light and love in the presence of Jesus.

HATHA YOGA – A method utilizing physical exercises to control the body and attain union of the self with God.

ISHVARA-PRANIDHANA – The path of surrendering to God. True freedom comes once you surrender yourself completely to God.

JNANA YOGA – The path of wisdom through the study of ancient texts and, even, self-study.

KAPHLABATI – A powerful cleansing and energizing type of breath exercise. The focus is on exhaling and simultaneously contracting the abdomen muscles with each powerful exhalation.

KARMA YOGA – The path of selfless service to others.

KOSHAS – These are five energetic layers that move from the outmost layer of the skin to the deep spiritual core. The five layers include the physical body, the pranic or subtle body, the deep recesses of the mind and emotions, the wisdom body, and, finally, into the pure and radiant bliss body.

MALA BEADS – A string of beads, usually 108 total, that are used for keeping count while reciting, chanting, or mentally repeating a mantra or prayer.

MANIPURA CHAKRA – The naval chakra is the seat of a person's sense of power and the ability to be confident and in-control of their lives.

MANTRA – A sacred sound, word or phrase believed to have psychological and spiritual meaning. A mantra may or may not have syntactic structure or literal meaning. It is a form of prayer.

MEDITATION – This is a precise technique for resting the mind and attaining a state of consciousness within. It is a science, which means that the process of meditation follows a particular order and produces results that brings oneness with God.

MUDRA – These are hand postures, commonly referred to as hand yoga, that are directly related to the energy flow in the human body. In Sanskrit, the word mudra means "closure" or "seal" meaning that mudras are used in a way to lock and guide energy through the body.

MULADHARA CHAKRA – The root chakra represents our foundation of feeling grounded. It governs our most basic survival needs.

NAMASTE – A word used at the end of a yoga practice while holding the palms together in front of the heart. It means "the light in me honors the light in you". Christians might add, "And together, we share the light of Christ to the world."

NI-YAMAS – These are five personal observances that relate to our inner world that include: saucha - purity/cleanliness; santosha - contentment; tapas - burning desire; svadhyaya - self-study/inner exploration; ishvara-pranidhana - surrender to God.

OM – This is a mystic syllable that is considered the most sacred sound and mantra. It can be chanted at the beginning and/or the end of yoga classes. The word has been referred to as "the sound of the universe". For Christian yoga, it is another way to end the class as if chanting Amen.

PRANAYAMA – This is the formal practice of controlling the breath, which is the source of the vital energy in the body.

PRATYAHARA – This is the practice of withdrawing from the senses. It can also defined as gaining mastery over external influences. By withdrawing from your senses, you turn inward.

RAJA YOGA – The most structured or "royal" path and includes the eight limbed progression. Raja yoga is the path that leads to union with God through the mental mastery of the mind, body, and breath. It calls upon the physical and mental disciple of the poses of Hatha Yoga.

SAHASWARA CHAKRA – The highest and seventh chakra, located at the crown of the head, represents the ability to be fully connected spiritually.

SAMADHI – An intense state of meditation, commonly referred to as the union or oneness with God. The eighth and final limb of yoga is connected to the crown chakra, where a shining, bright light stems from the top of your head and reaches up to the heavens to God. Samadhi urges you to escape from worldly troubles and enter into your original innocent self of pure joy. There you will bask in the brightness of the Lord.

SANSKRIT – An Indo-European, Indic language, in use since 1200 B.C.E. as the religious and classical literary language of India.

SANTOSHA – The principle of contentment and having the ability to feel satisfied within the present moment.

SATYA – This is the discipline of truth and the avoidance of all lies, exaggeration and pretense.

SAUCHA – The principle of cleanliness and purity in body, mind, and environment so that a higher quality of life can be experienced.

SUN SALUTATIONS – In Sanskrit, Surya Namaskar, or Sun Salutations is a series of postures performed in a single, graceful flow. Each movement is coordinated with the breath. Inhale as you extend or stretch, and exhale as you fold or contract.

SVADHISHTANA CHAKRA – The sacral chakra is the seat of creativity, joy, enthusiasm, sexuality, and sensuality.

SWADHYAYA – This is the discipline of self-study. It is an inward journey in order to truly learn about ourselves.

TAPAS – The burning desire of an individual to find their own personal passions or life's purpose. It is the willingness to do what is necessary to reach the goal.

VISHUDDHA CHAKRA – The throat chakra is the seat of communication and truth.

YAMAS – There are five self-regulating restraints involving our interactions with other people and the world at large. These include: ahimsa - nonviolence; satya - truthfulness; asteya - non-stealing; brahmacharya - moderation (often interpreted as sexual purity); aparigraha - non-greediness.

YOGA SUTRAS – The classic Sutras (thought-threads), compiled over 1500 years ago by Sage Patanjali, cover the yogic teachings on ethics, meditation, and physical postures, and provide directions for dealing with situations in daily life.

ABOUT THE AUTHOR

Sally Bassett, Ph.D., E-RYT 500

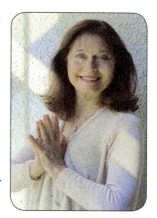

Sally's enthusiasm toward life as well as her creative and spiritual approach to yoga have been keys to her success. She is an adjunct professor at both Butler University, teaching yoga basics and philosophy, and at the Christian Theological Seminary, teaching "yoga and spirituality". Sally continues to teach at Peace through Yoga studios, which she originally founded in 2002.

Sally is also president and founder of Peace through Yoga Foundation, a nonprofit organization where the mission is to make an impact through transformational yoga and service. The service, or karma yoga, is accomplished through the foundation's International Center for Girls in the heart of the Costa Rican rainforest area. Sally leads week-long retreats there that include yoga, adventure, and service.

Sally has traveled to over 140 countries and has held numerous positions from flight attendant to C.E.O. She went from the galley to the boardroom during her thirty years in the travel industry. Some trips eventually evolved to a mixture of volunteering and tourism (a concept she helped coin called "voluntourism"). She completed her doctorate degree at Purdue University in tourism with the emphasis on international humanitarian work.

Sally's desire has been to make more of an impact with global sustainable projects on trips offered. Projects have included helping build a birthing center and an elementary school in Uganda, supporting a children's home in India, and a preschool in Kenya, and currently operating the International Center for Girls in Costa Rica through her foundation.

Sally lives on a horse farm in Indiana with her husband, Dennis, and delights in her three adult children, their spouses, and a grand-daughter named Olivia.